C000121099

Glucose Control Eating©

Lose Weight Stay Slimmer
Live Healthier Live Longer

By Rick Mystrom

Acknowledged Diabetes and Weight-Loss Authority

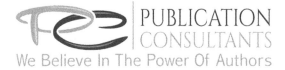

PUBLICATION CONSULTANTS
We Believe In The Power Of Authors

PO Box 221974 Anchorage, Alaska 99522-1974
books@publicationconsultants.com—www.publicationconsultants.com

ISBN: 978-1-59433-719-2

eBook ISBN Number: 978-1-59433-720-8

Library of Congress Number: 2017945479

Library of Congress Catalog Card Number: 2021924720

Manufactured in the United States of America

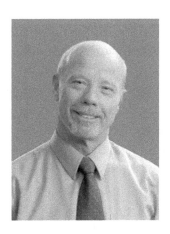

Other books by Rick Mystrom

My Wonderful Life with Diabetes

What Should I Eat? to Solve Diabetes,
Lose Weight, and Live Healthy
Your Type 2 Diabetes Lifeline.

About the Author

Rick Mystrom was diagnosed with Type 1 diabetes in 1964 while attending the University of Colorado at Boulder. Instead of denying the reality that was diabetes, he chose to shape that reality into living a healthy, bold, and active life with diabetes and added a promise to never complain about having diabetes.

In 1972 Rick and his young family moved to Alaska, where he started and operated two successful businesses. Nine years after moving to Alaska, he was named Alaska's Small Businessperson of the Year and one of America's top three small businessmen.

He served two terms on the Anchorage Assembly and was elected to two terms as mayor of Anchorage. He was elected chairman of the Alaska Conference of Mayors and was twice selected as Alaska's Elected Official of the Year. He also served as chairman of America's Olympic Bid Committee for the 1992 and 1994 Olympic Winter Games.

At 78 years of age, and having diabetes for 58 years, Rick Mystrom is a paragon of good health. His last stress test categorized him as equivalent to an active person 26 years younger than his actual age. He credits his good health to good eating habits, an active lifestyle, and an understanding of foods. For more than 40 years, he has tested his blood 5 to 10 times a day and has a unique understanding of which foods contribute to good health and which detract from good health.

For the past 10 years, Rick has meticulously measured, organized, and graphed—in a way never before done—the impact of different foods and combinations of foods on blood glucose and weight gain or loss.

Mystrom has used this information as a core of his books on healthy eating for diabetics. While his readers gratefully share how they have lowered their blood glucose, rid themselves of the need for diabetes medications, and feel much better, they rave about how much weight they have lost by learning how to control their blood glucose.

In this latest book, Mystrom beautifully organizes and explains Glucose Control Eating©, not as a diet, but as a lifetime eating style.

For American adults who are anywhere between slightly overweight and obese, this book is your answer to a longer, healthier, more enjoyable life.

Table of Contents

Preface

"Forty-two percent of Americans put on unwanted weight during the COVID shutdown. That, by itself, grabs attention. But more worrisome is that 48% of younger Americans, ages 25 to 40, put on weight—with a stunning average gain of 41 pounds."

— *The Week Magazine*, April 23, 2021 —

Even before the COVID shutdown, more than one-third of Americans were classified as overweight and another third were classified by the CDC as obese. More and more medical professionals and researchers now use 70% as the total number of overweight and obese Americans.

Those startling numbers combined with the CDC's data showing that obesity is the second leading risk factor for death among those hospitalized with COVID, have quietly got the attention of millions of overweight Americans.

But for most folks who are overweight or obese, the real issue is quality of life. They would like to feel better, move better, and look better—wouldn't we all. That's what this book is all about. It's not just about losing weight; it's about living slimmer, living healthier, and living a long, good-quality life.

People all over the United States are ready to try to take off the unwanted weight they gained. They're ready to start walking, jogging, riding bikes, taking exercise classes, walking the malls, or just moving more outside. They're hoping to lose the weight they have gained. But they'll fail, mostly.

Just moving and increasing activity isn't going to cause much weight loss. People cannot outwork bad eating habits. For typical

Americans—not competitive athletes—what you put into your mouth is about 80% of weight gain or weight loss; how you burn it is the other 20%. Many doctors, medical professionals and their odd bedfellows, bodybuilders, generally concur with that statement. I explain in this book how I've come to the same conclusion through testing.

Most people don't know how to lose weight. They try different diets with good intentions and hope. They fail. They try again and fail. Then they often give up and return to eating for satisfaction and fulfillment.

Why have so many failed? They've tried cutting out sweets. That helps but it's only part of the cause of their weight gain They've tried counting calories. That's burdensome and again only part of the story. They've failed because no one has ever told them in clear, everyday terms, how we all gain and lose weight.

Most weight-loss books are written by smart, well-intentioned people who read a lot of other weight-loss books and write their own book based on their collected 2nd hand knowledge and their personal experience.

This is the very reason so many weight-loss books focus on counting calories. But counting calories hasn't worked for Americans. Although calories are now listed on almost all packaged foods. It's made no difference. America's weight bulge continues and has even accelerated.

This book is different. It's based on more than 40 years of empirical testing and more than 85,000 tests on the impact of foods and drinks on weight.

How We Gain and Lose Weight

To understand how we gain and lose weight, we need to start with insulin. Medical researchers and internal medicine doctors almost universally agree that the amount of insulin a person produces is the determiner of weight gain and weight loss. Gary Taubes, a medical researcher and recipient of multiple awards from the National Association of Science Writers, refers to insulin as "the stop-and-go light of weight gain and loss."

Produce more insulin—you will gain weight. Produce less insulin—you will lose weight.

Insulin is a hormone that allows the glucose (also called blood sugar) in your blood to get out of your bloodstream and into your cells for energy for whatever your current activity or inactivity is. If you have more glucose in your bloodstream than your current energy need, the excess is stored in your liver (called glycogen in its storage form). If your liver is full and you still have excess glucose in your bloodstream, the rest is stored as body fat around your butt, your thighs, your belly—and generally every place you don't want it to be.

How do you control the amount of insulin your body produces?

You do it by controlling the amount of glucose you put into your bloodstream. Put in less glucose, your body will produce less insulin and you will lose weight. Put in more glucose, your body will produce more insulin and you will gain weight. That brings us to the premise of this book: *Control your blood glucose and you control your weight.*

- Lower blood glucose and you will lose weight.
  This is universal.

- How do you lower your blood glucose?
  The answers are in this book.

What Foods Create Blood Glucose?

Blood glucose is not created just by sweets—it's created by all foods. Proteins create glucose, fats create glucose, vegetables create glucose, fruits create glucose, fruit juices create glucose, starchy foods create glucose, and of course, sweets create glucose. The key to losing weight is to consume less of the foods (including drinks) that create large amounts of glucose and replace them with foods and drinks that create smaller amounts of glucose *and* go into the bloodstream more slowly.

This is true of everyone. People may burn foods differently but the creation of glucose from all foods is the same, varying only by the size of the person and the resulting different volume of blood circulating in people of different sizes.

Why Is It So Hard to Lose Weight?

Body fat is hard to lose because the body automatically burns the easiest source of energy first—blood glucose; when blood glucose gets too low, the body then uses the next easiest source of energy—glycogen in the liver—which converts back to glucose and goes into the bloodstream. Then and only then, after the liver is depleted of glycogen, does the body begin to use body fat. That is why body fat is so hard to get rid of. It's the last source of energy used and is also a very stable molecule that is hard to break down.

You can gain weight easily, simply by putting more glucose in your bloodstream than you need for your current activity or inactivity. But it's harder to lose weight because body fat is the last source of energy your body uses. This is the very reason that you can gain weight quickly, but losing weight takes longer.

If insulin is the weight loss stop-and-go signal, the question then becomes: How can you reduce the amount of insulin your body produces so your weight gain stops, and your weight loss starts, and continues until you reach your desired weight?

You control the amount of glucose you put into your bloodstream. Put in less glucose, your body will produce less insulin and you will lose weight. Put in more glucose, your body will produce more insulin and you will gain weight. That brings us back to the premise of this book.

Control your glucose and you control your weight.

How do you control your glucose and your weight? How can you know which foods create lots of glucose and weight gain and which foods create less glucose and weight loss?

In this book, I will not only tell you. I will show you.

Why Am I Uniquely Qualified to Tell You and Show You How to Lower Your Blood Glucose and Lose Weight?

I was diagnosed with Type 1 diabetes when I was 20. I am now 78 years old and very healthy.

Because I am a Type 1 diabetic, my pancreas doesn't balance my blood glucose as it does in nondiabetics. I must continually balance my blood glucose myself. To master that balancing act and live the long, healthy, and productive life I am living, I have embraced the challenge of controlling my blood glucose and maintaining a healthy weight by testing, recording, and graphing my own blood glucose. I started by testing four or five times a day. Now I test 10 to 15 times a day. I estimate that I have given myself more than 85,000 blood glucose tests and counting over the past 40 years.

I have tested multiple times before and after nearly every meal I've eaten and many times after snacks as well. I also measure before and after exercise so I can assess how the glucose created by food I have eaten is burned.

I have had to learn how to control my blood glucose to avoid the devastating consequences and short life span of poorly controlled diabetes. My exceptional health and ideal weight are the beneficial side effects of learning which meals will create high blood glucose and weight gain and which meals will create low blood glucose and weight loss.

———

Today I'm one of the longest-living, healthy Type 1 diabetics in America. I've had Type 1 diabetes for 58 years and have no health issues. My last stress test categorized me as equivalent to an active person 26 years younger than my actual age. I'm not a dedicated workout guy; but I am an active person who has had to learn how to eat well or die early. I chose the former. It's paid off in good health and an active, healthy, fun, quality of life as I approach 80. On my website, rickmystrom.com, you can see some of my activities in my mid to late '70s.

I've accomplished a lot while living with Type 1 diabetes. I was mayor of Anchorage for most of the 1990s, a successful businessman recognized in a White House Rose Garden ceremony as one of the three top small-business people in America; was chairman of America's Winter Olympic bids from 1985 to1989, and I've coached 20 youth sports teams.

But more than just living productively with diabetes, I have learned what to eat, when to eat, and how to eat to live slim, live healthy, and live long.

Here is a story I tell in many of the hundred or so speeches I have given about blood glucose control:

> About 25 years after I was first diagnosed with diabetes, I told a doctor that I thought I was healthier because I had diabetes than I would have been without diabetes. I will never forget his response. He said firmly and without hesitation, "I doubt it." That was discouraging but I don't recall letting it bother me much.
>
> About 10 years later I said the same thing to another doctor. His comment was a little more encouraging, "Well, you look pretty good, maybe." I was making progress.
>
> Then about eight years later at a reception, I was talking to two doctors who knew me, or at least knew of me. When I told them I thought I was healthier because I was a 50-year diabetic than I would have been if I hadn't had diabetes, they both reacted the same way, "Rick, write a book. Tell America what you've done. Millions of people need that help. Do it."

I did. I wrote three books on healthy eating and living for diabetics. Now I'm writing this book for all those who would like to lose weight in a very healthy way and live slimmer and healthier for the rest of their lives. It's also written with those people in mind who may be satisfied with their weight now but want to avoid the age-related weight creepage that is so common in America.

———

In order to share this information on controlling blood glucose with the 30 million Type 2 diabetics in the United States and the estimated 30 million borderline diabetics, as well as the 3 million Type 1 diabetics, I have charted and graphed many of these tests and published them in two of the books I have written about blood glucose control for diabetics:

What Should I Eat? to Solve Diabetes, Lose Weight, and Live Healthy and *Your Type 2 Diabetes Lifeline.* My third book is a memoir of living with Type 1 diabetes, titled, *My Wonderful Life with Diabetes.*

The life-changing stories I've received from diabetics, prediabetics, and borderline diabetics have been very fulfilling and touching, but quite honestly—I expected these results. What has surprised me, though, is the volume of stories, texts, and effusive comments I have received about *how much weight the readers of the two books on glucose control have lost.*

If you would like to lose weight and keep it off in a healthy and permanent way, reading this book and applying this information will not only make your pounds melt away but will also improve your mobility, your quality of life, and your appearance.

Foreword

By Thomas S. Nighswander, MD MPH

Rick Mystrom and his family moved to Anchorage in the same year my wife and I did—1972. But it was not until the company he started, Mystrom Advertising, had been in existence for several years that I started to hear references to him as an emerging public figure of some stature. This was an underestimation!

Looking at his leadership in the dramatic transformations of Anchorage and Alaska in the '80s and '90s, one begins to understand his inspirations, motivations, style, and philosophy of service.

To really know what makes Rick tick, you must understand a bit about diabetes and his trials and errors over the years in not only surviving the disease, but even thriving because of it.

His diabetes weaves in and out of stories about both his public and private life. On balance, he says, it has been a positive influence and, in fact, he probably would not be as healthy as he is today if he had not had diabetes.

His diagnosis of insulin-dependent Type 1 diabetes 58 years ago at age 20 was a clarion call for him to understand his disease and take charge of his health. He wins the gold medal in both these categories.

As Rick's story unfolds, I am struck by several recurring themes: attitude, management, and a passionate desire to understand the impact of foods and combinations of foods on blood glucose and weight, and to share that information with others.

Rick has become so expert at controlling blood glucose that many members of the Anchorage medical community use his advice and his books to help their patients lower blood glucose and lose weight.

Griff Steiner, a nationally respected ophthalmologist, captured the value of Rick's positive attitude in this comment published in Rick's first book, *My Wonderful Life with Diabetes*:

> I believe the overwhelming message of Rick's book is how priceless a positive attitude is in living a great life. Rick's optimism clearly played a dramatic role in his many successes, including how well he has managed a potentially devastating disease. As an ophthalmologist, I have never seen anyone with Type 1 diabetes without any evidence of eye damage after a few decades, let alone more than 50 years after diagnosis. Rick's story is an example for anyone, diabetic or not, to take charge of the challenges in life rather than letting them take charge of you.
>
> Griff Steiner, MD, Ophthalmology

Beyond his positive attitude, Rick's passion for managing diabetes by testing, recording, and graphing the impact of foods on his blood sugar has been instrumental in his health. Rick has tested his own blood sugar more than 10 times a day since self-testing first became available to the public.

The results and graphs of these tests have become the core of Rick's second book, *What Should I Eat to solve diabetes, lose weight, and live healthy*, and his third book, *Your Type 2 Diabetes Lifeline*.

These books have been embraced by many in the medical community in Alaska and are commonplace in waiting rooms and exam rooms throughout Anchorage.

Here are some comments about them from medical professionals in Alaska:

> "Please send me two more boxes of your books. I am passionate about your message. I give them to the resident physicians in my classes and to my patients."
>
> **Murray Buttner, M.D.**
> Faculty, Alaska Family Medicine Residency
> Anchorage, Alaska

"Your books are so helpful I keep them in exam rooms, with pages highlighted for my patients to read before I come in to talk with them about my recommended approach to dealing with their diabetes by eating properly. You should also expect more book orders; I'm presenting on Type 2 diabetes next week at the Society of Rural Physicians of Canada's annual medical conference and the success of your book will be highlighted in my presentation."

Dr. Peter J. Montesano
Family Practice Specialist
Anchorage, Alaska

From Rick's endocrinologist of 40 years:

"Rick Mystrom never let diabetes prevent him from accomplishing everything he wanted in life: good health, success in business, community service, family, and politics. Rick Mystrom knew that understanding his disease was crucial to his health. He is the most knowledgeable person living with diabetes in my extensive practice and frequently serves as a role model and authoritative resource for others."

Jeanne R. Bonar MD, FACP, FACE
Endocrinology, Internal Medicine

"If every newly diagnosed diabetic, regardless of type, would adopt Rick's two premises: having a positive attitude about living with diabetes and taking personal responsibility for modifying your food intake …the improvement in the quality of life would be outstanding."

Sue Sampson, RN, BSN
Anchorage, Alaska

"I've been reading books on diabetes since 1974. Your book is the best written book on diabetes I have ever found. After I read your book, I bought four more to loan out to members of my church and one to donate to my hometown library."

R. Clinch, RN BSN
Wasilla, Alaska

As you can tell, Rick has earned the support of many in the Alaskan medical community. But even more, Rick is a role model for diabetic patients and for those in public service. One will find his motivations are clear and altruistic. He has been driven by what he thinks will best improve the lives and well-being of those who have elected him to public office. His enthusiasm for life is infectious. His positive attitude has carried him and others to achievements they never thought possible.

Having had Type 1 diabetes for over half century has not prevented Rick from taking on any challenge, whether it was in his public role, the variety of sports competitions he loves, or in other adventures and a few misadventures throughout his very full life.

Now Rick has taken on another challenge—dealing with the largest controllable epidemic in America today: obesity. In this book, *Glucose Control Eating©*, Rick applies what he has learned from more than 85,000 self-administered blood glucose tests to clearly and simply show which foods will cause big increases in blood glucose and weight gain and which foods will cause small increases in blood glucose and result in weight loss.

In Rick's previous books on controlling blood sugar (glucose) and reversing Type 2 diabetes, he has received many stories about how Type 2 diabetics have lowered their blood sugars and are now off their diabetes medications. But more common than the stories on lowered blood glucose are the stories about how much weight readers have lost.

In Rick's new book, featuring Glucose Control Eating©, Rick explains the dominant role blood glucose plays in weight gain and loss.

He explains, in simple terms, how we gain and lose weight and why the determining factor of weight gain or loss is blood glucose.

He explains why counting calories hasn't worked for Americans.

He explains why the advice to "cut back on carbs" is too vague and that carbs should be broken into four subcategories based on how much they raise blood glucose, and therefore how much they impact weight gain.

He doesn't just tell you *what* foods and combinations of foods you should eat to lose weight, he wants you to *understand why* those foods will help you lose weight.

He very deftly and convincingly leads you to your own conclusion that if you lower your blood glucose, you will lose weight.

In conclusion, Rick has such a unique and detailed understanding of blood glucose control that he can simply look at a plate of food and adjust his insulin input with astounding accuracy. He's used that expertise to improve the lives of many of his fellow Alaskans.

In his new book, *Glucose Control Eating©*, he is applying this knowledge to help the two thirds of American adults who are overweight or obese.

Rick is the expert. I am the learner.

Thomas S. Nighswander MD MPH
Professor of Family Medicine
Assistant Clinical Dean,
Alaska WWAMI* Program
for the School of Medicine
University of Washington
Anchorage, Alaska

---

* Note: WWAMI is the abbreviation of the cooperative medical degree program representing Washington, Wyoming, Alaska, Montana, and Idaho.

Introduction

What You Will Learn from This Book

I am writing this book on weight loss because of weight readers have lost after reading one or both of my first books on glucose control. The enthusiastic weight-loss success folks have experienced after reading those books compels me to directly address the issue of unwanted weight and obesity experienced by more than two thirds of American adults.

In this book you won't just learn *what to eat*, but you'll learn *why*.

You will learn in ordinary, day-to-day language how your body gains weight and how it loses weight.

You will learn why America's obesity epidemic started five years after the introduction of *The Food Pyramid*—just long enough for Americans to start following its recommendations and seeing the results.

Americans started eating the suggested way and saw the results on their bathroom scales. The results weren't good. The growth in obesity started and continues to this day even after the Food Pyramid was changed—without much fanfare—to the *My Plate* recommendations. Those eating recommendations are better but still not good for avoiding weight gain or losing weight.

You will learn that blood glucose is the determining factor in weight gain and loss.

You will learn that all foods—not just sweets—create blood glucose.

You will learn that the key to losing weight is to eat less of the high-glucose-creating foods and more of the low-glucose-creating foods.

You will learn visually from the graphs in this book which foods create the most blood glucose and which create the least blood glucose.

You will learn why counting calories hasn't worked for Americans.

You will learn why the advice to "cut carbs" is too vague and why I break carbs into four distinct sub-groups based on their impact on blood glucose and weight. When those groups are added to protein and fat, you will have *six food groups instead of just three* to make your weight loss much easier.

You will learn that fat is a friend of weight loss—but not always. When eaten alone or combined with certain foods, fat does not make you fat; but combined with certain other foods it does. That is why I call fat a *conditional friend* of weight loss.

You will learn which foods you can combine fat with to lose weight and which foods that combined with fat will cause weight gain.

You will learn that as little as 15 minutes of moderate activity, like walking, between the time you finish dinner and the time you go to bed will have a measurable impact on weight loss.

You will learn, not only what changes to make in your eating habits, but also *how* to make those changes.

In summary, you will learn how to lose weight the healthy way… and how to maintain the new, healthier you.

I have learned all of this through my passion for blood glucose testing and analyzing the results of more than 85,000 blood tests I've given myself over the past 40+ years.

The Breakthroughs in This Book

This book introduces Glucose Control Eating©, an eating lifestyle that is easy to maintain for the rest of your life. This book is unique for many reasons. Here are but a few.

1. This book demonstrates clearly that the determining force behind weight gain and weight loss is the amount of glucose you put in your bloodstream.

2. This book clearly and unequivocally illustrates that blood glucose (sugar) does not come just from eating sweets but comes from every type of food we eat, proteins, fats, and carbohydrates.

3. Glucose Control Eating© is based on never-before-published empirical research on tests that only a healthy, motivated, long-term Type 1 diabetic can do. The results show not only how *individual foods* impact blood glucose and therefore weight but also—for the first time ever—how certain *combinations of foods (meals)* impact blood glucose and weight gain or weight loss.

4. This book, for the first time, *breaks food into six food groups* instead of just the standard three food groups—proteins, fats, and carbohydrates. Protein and fat remain as categories, but carbohydrates (carbs) are broken into four distinct sub-groups: *sweet carbs, starchy carbs, fruit carbs, and vegetable carbs,* based on their impact on blood glucose and weight. Add those four to protein and fat and you have six groups of foods that all impact blood glucose and weight differently.

5. This book clearly illustrates, for the first time, *why counting calories* has not worked for America. It graphically shows how foods in different groups but with the same number of calories will have a dramatically different effect on blood glucose and weight gain or loss.

6. This book also illustrates that *you do not have to starve yourself to lower your blood glucose and lose weight*; you will never win the war against hunger, and you don't have to. You just eat more of the foods that cause a smaller, slower rise in blood glucose and less of the foods that cause a bigger rise in blood glucose.

7. This book addresses for the first time how foods react differently when combined with other foods. This is an essential principle to understand. After all, we eat most meals as combinations of foods.

8. This book also demonstrates for the first time that the standard advice for borderline or Type 2 diabetics on blood sugar and weight control is not wrong, but *backward*. That advice is, to avoid or reverse Type 2 diabetes, "you must lose weight to lower your blood glucose." This book demonstrates clearly and convincingly that the better advice is, "First, lower your blood glucose, then you will lose weight."

The old advice suggests you should deal with the effect (losing weight) first and then the cause (lower your blood glucose). My advice is deal with the cause first—lower your blood glucose, and then the effect—losing weight— will follow.

For all the above reasons, Glucose Control Eating© is a groundbreaking book that will improve the health and lives of millions of Americans.

Understand and Remember This:

- You *can't* win in a fight against hunger.

- You *can't* lose weight by cutting way back on eating and being hungry all the time.

- You *can* lose weight by eating more of the right foods and less of the wrong foods.

Which foods are right, and which are wrong?

The answers are in this book.

Testimonials

Sample Comments on Presentations

By Rick Mystrom

"Rick Mystrom was a terrific speaker.
He had great clarity in his presentation.
It was personal, practical, and enjoyable."

"Number seven speaker, (Mystrom), was wonderful."

"I enjoyed Rick Mystrom. He was very
encouraging and upbeat."

"Please repeat Rick Mystrom's *What Should I Eat* presentation.

We missed it and were told it was excellent."

"Really liked the mayor from Alaska, Rick Mystrom"

"Rick Mystrom was the best." "Excellent." "Awesome"

"I like surprises. Rick Mystrom's *What Should I Eat*,
presentation was a delightful surprise."

"When you have speakers like Rick, who have so much
to share, please allow them more time."

"I've been a nurse for 32 years. This was the best
presentation on healthy eating I've ever seen."

Sample Comments on Rick Mystrom's Books from Medical Professionals

"Rick Mystrom never let diabetes prevent him from accomplishing everything he wanted in life: good health, success in business, community service, family, and politics. Rick Mystrom knew that understanding his disease was crucial to his health. He has become the most knowledgeable person living with diabetes in my extensive practice and frequently serves as a role model and authoritative resource for others."

Jeanne R. Bonar, MD
Endocrinology, Internal Medicine

"Rick's story is an example for anyone, diabetic or not, to take charge of the challenges in life rather than letting them take charge of you."

Griff Steiner MD
Ophthalmology
Anchorage, Alaska

"If every newly diagnosed diabetic, regardless of type, could adopt Rick's two premises: having a positive attitude about living with diabetes and taking personal responsibility for modifying your food intake…the improvement in the quality of life would be outstanding

Sue Sampson, RN, BSN
Anchorage, Alaska

"I commend you for taking the time to document all your personal food reactions to show the downside of hi-carb foods. Your book should be a best-seller!"

Pat DeVoe, RN, BSN
Diabetes Action Research and Education Foundation
Bethesda, MD

"I've been reading books on diabetes and healthy eating since 1974. Your book is the best written book on those subjects I have ever found. After I read your book, I bought four more copies to loan out to members of my church."

R. Clinch, RN BSN
Wasilla, Alaska

"Your books are going like hotcakes down here. We need them for an upcoming health event. Could we please get another box? I am very passionate about your message!

You are doing so much to help people with diabetes and obesity. The medical world is mismanaging this epidemic. Keep it up!

Thank you."

W. Murray Buttner, MD
Faculty, Alaska Family Medicine Residency

"Rick, your books are an integral part of my practice. Each exam room has a copy of What Should I Eat, well-creased to the graphs of shrimp versus pasta. On an average day I am using your graphs at least four times to offer people an approach to eating without telling them exactly what to eat. I find your approach to work well."

Peter Montesano, MD
Family Practice
Anchorage, Alaska

Sample Comments from Readers

"I heard you speak on diabetes and bought your book. Twenty pounds gone, off diabetes meds and blood pressure meds, no more Tums. THANK YOU, and God Bless You."

Robert Maxon
Anchorage

"I can't say enough about how your book helped me and my husband. We turn the TV off and read it out loud together. I've lost 45 pounds and my husband has lost 15 pounds."

Laura
Colorado

"Thanks to Rick Mystrom, I've changed my eating style and lost 34 pounds. It wasn't fast but it was steady and easy to keep off. I'm off all my medications now except for one. Thank you, Mr. Mystrom."

Rabbi Greenberg
Anchorage

"Rick, A few months ago, a new patient came in for a physical, he was an older man with coronary heart disease and high blood sugars. He was also quite overweight. I told him about your book and gave him a copy. Yesterday he called me to tell me he had lost 65 pounds and his blood sugars were near normal. He was leaving for vacation. I told him to call me when he comes back so we can celebrate what he has done."

Murray Buttner MD

"I want you to know, Rick, that your advice saved my father's life. Thank you. Thank you. Thank you."

Denise Trutonic
Anchorage

"I have referred to your book countless times. I have lost 20 pounds so far and it is the easiest weight I have ever lost. All the other calorie restriction diets were white-knuckle events. You are spot on!! I have shared your book with several friends. Thank you so much."

Anon. (by request)

"I have been following your diet recommendations (with occasional bad days). My weight is down 40 pounds and for the first time in 30 years all my bloodwork is in the normal range. My 90-day blood sugars are normal, liver enzymes low normal, total cholesterol down, good cholesterol up. Thank you, thank you, thank you, Rick."

Chuck C.
Anchorage

"Your book, *What Should I Eat*, is so well written and understandable. It is the best book I've ever read on healthy eating and diabetes. As soon as I finished it, I went out and bought another book for a friend. Now I keep going back to your book and I'm doing great now."

Carol Childs
Anchorage, AK

"I have been a Type 2 diabetic for almost 16 years and insulin-dependent for about half that time. The graphs [in Rick Mystrom's book, *What Should I Eat*] are the first of their kind I have ever seen and bring an "ah ha" moment in understanding the effect of (certain) carbohydrates on glucose levels. I highly recommend this book."

John Eckheard
Pomona, CA

"I saw Rick on TV and his message really clicked with me. I am not diabetic but have struggled with my weight all my life. This is by far the most detailed and intelligent explanation of the ill effects of bad carbs on weight gain I have ever seen. I have followed his eating plan for two weeks and have already lost 9 pounds, but best of all, I have the knowledge to understand why I need to eat this way for health and to avoid diabetes. Thank you, Rick."

Melinda M. Hofstad

"I've been reading your book. I LOVE IT. I will never look at food the same way again. I've already lost 7 pounds. It was so easy to lose I fully expect I will never regain that weight and will lose more."

Kathleen Madden
Anchorage

"Your book is well written, concise, and to the point, especially the graphs and illustrations to promote a healthy eating lifestyle. I take pride that an Alaskan has made such a contribution. I am recommending your book to my family and friends. Thank you for your contribution to my ongoing battle not to become a diabetic and to control my weight."

William M. (Bill) Bankston
Anchorage, AK

"Having my Dr. tell me that I might have diabetes really woke me up. I knew I needed help. Rick Mystrom's book, What Should I Eat from the start was clear, to the point, and extremely informative. Who would have thought a book about a disease would be so engaging! I never skipped a page."

Robert Herndon
Roseville, CA

"As parents of a recently diagnosed Type 1 diabetes son, Rick Mystrom's book has not only profoundly impacted his diet but has changed the rest of our family's approach to food. Rick has given us a major contribution that will improve the American diet, leading to a higher quality of life for all.

Thank you, Rick!"

Bill and Jean Bredar
Anchorage, AK

"Bravo!...A powerful message that will help so many people— now and forever.

Well done!"

Malcom Roberts
Author, Alaskan Leader

"Your book has sprouted wings and is flying off the shelves."

Sally McCollor
Providence Hospital Gift Shop
Anchorage, AK

"I bought your book and within days started feeling results. I have come back to buy a copy for my sister. Thank you!"

Sam
Anchorage, Alaska

"Diabetes never stopped Rick Mystrom from doing all the things he wanted to do. His life story and amazing success along the way demonstrates how someone with a positive outlook [who] works hard, can succeed regardless of the challenges he faced."

Bill Fedderson
Anchorage

"This book is not just for diabetics but for all who are interested in good health and weight loss. I purchased it from my local bookstore. I am not diabetic but need to lose weight so I thought I would give it a try. I found it to be very informative. It has given me a new prospective on 'dieting' and not regaining all the weight back."

Amazon Customer
5 stars

"Mr. Mystrom has lived wonderfully with Type 1 diabetes for his 70+ years. In this book, he explains in layman's language how insulin is produced as a response to the foods we eat. He graphed results from the hundreds—more likely thousands—of readings to track how fast individual foods raise glucose levels. If you want to avoid diabetes, or just lose weight, this book is inspirational. I don't know why the medical associations haven't picked up on his research, but, for the sake of their patients, they should!"

Amazon Customer
5 stars

"The easiest and most informative book I have ever read about controlling my diabetes and weight. This really works and believe me I have tried everything."

Amazon Customer
5 stars

Chapter 1

America's Overweight Bulge

You are not alone in your fight to lose weight. The advice initiated by Congress in the late '70s, published by the Department of Agriculture, promoted by a compliant media, taught by well-intentioned educators nationwide, and reacted to by the grocery industry, has become an accepted standard for eating for more than a generation of Americans.

America's obesity epidemic started a few years after the Food Pyramid was first published and heavily promoted as the guide to healthy eating. Americans gained weight by doing what they were told.

It's important to note that it's not just the eating guidelines from the US government, the Food Pyramid, or its successor, My Plate, that caused the bulging of America's waistline. It's also how we don't categorize foods based on impact on weight, how we think measuring calories is the best way to control weight, and how we don't understand or consider the impact of foods when combined with other foods.

Additionally, the increases in sedentary behavior catalyzed by the big increases in television-watching time starting in the last half of the 20ᵗʰ century and the increase in computer, tablet, and smart-phone

---

AUTHOR'S NOTE:
Throughout this book, the language is simple and nontechnical, designed to promote your understanding of weight loss through healthy eating. It is also important to repeat the point that blood sugar and blood glucose are used interchangeably in the United States. I use the term blood glucose in this book because it more scientifically reflects what is contained in your blood.

screen time in the first two decades of the 2000s are certainly contributing factors.

Some Background on Our Country's Weight Bulge

Most weight-loss books are written by smart, well-intentioned people. Some are nutritionists, some are fitness buffs, some are medical doctors, and others have a passion for reading scores of books and articles on healthy eating and restructuring the information based on their own interests and theories.

America's problem is that the core resource used for teaching, studying, and writing about nutrition for nearly two generations has been guidance from the US Department of Agriculture . . . and that guidance is flawed.

The US Department of Agriculture's guidance for healthy eating was the result of the work of the Senate Select Committee on American Dietary Habits chaired by Senator George McGovern.

The conclusions of that committee in 1977 became the basis for the creation of the Government's guidance in what it thought and stated to be healthy eating habits.

Those conclusions got a public profile in 1984 with the creation of the *Food Wheel: A Pattern for Daily Food Choices.* The Food Wheel first visually promoted the position that a healthy day of meals should include 6 to 11 portions of the bread, cereal, rice, and pasta groups, but only a tiny bit of fat.

By 1992 that eating guidance was represented by the highly publicized and much better known *Food Pyramid.* The Food Pyramid had the same guidance of 6 to 11 portions of the bread, cereal, rice, and pasta groups a day and only a tiny bit of fat, but in a more easily grasped pyramid form instead of the earlier *Food Wheel.*

It took about five years for this eating guidance to start showing results. But the results were not good. In 1984, after about five years of promoting and teaching these recommendations, America's obesity epidemic as well as our Type 2 diabetes epidemic began.

Now, more than a generation later, more than two thirds of Americans are overweight and more than half of those folks are classified as obese. Concurrently, about 30 million Americans contracted Type 2 diabetes, with another 30 million estimated to be borderline diabetic. This happened in large part because we did what we were told.

By 2011, the USDA finally—but very quietly—admitted The Food Pyramid was wrong and changed to what it called "My Plate"—better, but still not effective for maintaining a healthy weight.

Even though the Federal Government replaced the Food Pyramid, it will still take another generation or so for America's eating habits to change and American grocers to react to those changes.

Since the Food Pyramid still influences America's daily food choices, we need to understand the problems it has foisted upon our eating habits.

What Were the Most Significant Problems with America's Eating Guidelines?

Two of the three significant flaws were incorrect major conclusions. The third flaw was one of understandable omission.

By the time you finish this book, you will understand these flaws and why Americans have gained so much weight since the promotion of this information. You will also understand, not only what to eat, but why.

The First Problem

The first and most impactfully wrong major conclusion was that Americans should eat 6 to 11 servings of the "bread, cereal, rice, and pasta group." That's right. *6 to 11 servings a day* of that group.

The cereal, bread, and pasta makers embraced that recommendation and the US and Canadian grain farmers responded by devoting more acreage to grains to meet the growing demand of the American consumers driven by the recommendations of the Food Pyramid. Grocers responded by devoting much more shelf space to those products.

As Americans responded by buying and eating more of that group of carbohydrates, the overweight bulge began.

The Second Problem

The *second incorrect major conclusion* was we were told to eat only a tiny amount of fat. We were told that fat is not a friend of good health. We were told *If you don't want to get fat, don't eat fat.*

What an easy sell that was to the American public. After all, fat has 9 calories per gram whereas protein and carbohydrates have only 5 calories per gram. Plus, dietary *fat* has the same name as body *fat*...and it feels the same. Push a finger on the fat on your arm, or around your hips, or stomach, and it feels the same as pushing your finger on the marbled fat of a rib-eye steak.

To meet Americans' desire to limit or even eliminate fat in their diets, the grocery industry responded with the creation and promotion of nonfat and low-fat foods. I presume profit was a motivation, but like the rest of America, the grocery industry likely believed low-fat and nonfat products were good for the health of their customers too. They bought into that idea just like the American public did.

In this book, you'll learn that fatty foods are a great friend of weight loss and improved good cholesterol (HDL) *if* they are eaten alone or with protein or vegetables in the same meal—think vegetable omelets, vegetables with butter, fish with fat-based sauces, and even fatty meat under certain conditions.

However, fat is a great contributor to weight gain and increased bad cholesterol if eaten with starchy carbs or sweet carbs in the same sitting, for example, butter with toast, pancakes, or waffles; or fatty meat with bread, rice, biscuits, or followed by a sweet dessert in the same meal.

Because my testing of the impact of fat in your diet is so different from what the American public has been told, and what the American public has done, I offer a lot more detail and recent evidence from medical researchers on fat, as well as my own research on fat, in coming chapters.

But first, the adjacent page a very visual illustration of the evolution of opinions on the role of fat in a healthy diet.

The Third Problem

The third problem with The Food Pyramid and its successor *My Plate* is the omission of what foods we should eat in combination with other foods to avoid weight gain. Clearly, we most often eat meals as combinations of foods, so how these foods impact your weight when they enter your bloodstream together is important.

It is very understandable that this was omitted. To my knowledge that subject had not been researched at that time or even today as far as I know.

The Evolution of Opinions on Fat

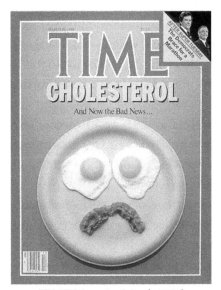

TIME *Magazine* March 1994

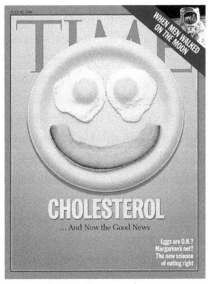

TIME *Magazine* July 1999

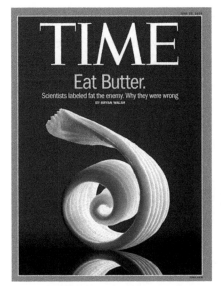

TIME *Magazine* June 2014

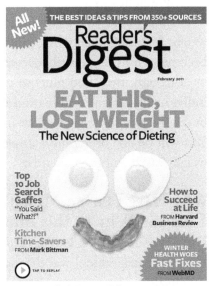

Reader's Digest February 2011

I have been doing research unknowingly on the impact of foods in combination with other foods throughout my 40 years of blood testing. It took me nearly 35 years to understand why my blood glucose was so easy to predict for single foods but so hard to predict for meals combining foods.

Sometimes the impact—on blood glucose and weight—of two foods being combined was greater than the sum of the impact of those foods separately and sometimes the sum of the impact was less than the impact of the two foods separately.

This is one of the more important revelations in my 40 years of testing and one of this book's important new breakthroughs for weight loss. You will see graphs in this book revealing which foods to combine and which foods not to combine for weight loss.

For example, you will see that fat is a friend of weight loss and contributor to good cholesterol (HDL) if eaten alone or with fish, eggs, and most vegetables. But it's a big contributor to weight gain and bad cholesterol (LDL) if eaten with any starchy carbs or sweet carbs in the same meal or within three hours after that meal with fat.

Understanding the conditional impact of eating fat is essential to healthy weight loss.

In this book, you will find graphs of foods that are promoters of weight loss individually but when combined with certain other foods become significant contributors to weight gain.

Through my blood glucose tests after eating thousands of foods individually and in combination with other foods, I know which combinations should be avoided or limited to lose weight and keep it off. This will be one of the most important new concepts to help you lose weight easily and permanently.

Why Have I Given Myself So Many Blood Glucose Tests and Why Is This Important to You?

I'm a Type 1 diabetic. Unlike Type 2 diabetes, Type 1 is not reversible, but it is manageable. I was diagnosed when I was 20. I'm now 78 and very healthy.

The credit for my good health belongs largely to the creators and developers of insulin pumps and glucose testers. They first became widely available about 40 years ago. Without those two inventions and their continual improvement in reliability and convenience, I can reasonably say I would not be alive today.

With those two tools, and a passion to live a long, healthy, and productive life with Type 1 diabetes, I have been able to maintain good control of my blood glucose.

It is important to state that I'm not an overzealous exerciser, but I am an active person who has participated in sports most of my life and who moves a lot during my normal daytime office activities. But my exceptional health has been overwhelmingly the result of learning what, how, and when to eat.

What I have learned about food from testing my blood glucose so often for more than 40 years has given me the knowledge and ability to stay healthy after 58 years with Type 1 diabetes.

I have shared the results of this testing in my first two books written for Type 2 diabetics or borderline diabetics.

The life-changing stories I have received from readers of these books have been very fulfilling. They talk excitedly about how they have lowered their blood glucose and are off all diabetic medications. I expected those results. What has surprised me, though, is the volume of stories, texts, emails, letters, and comments I have received about how much weight the readers of these two books have lost.

The feedback I get from so many of those who have read my books on glucose control seems to follow two patterns. The first pattern is something like this, *Your book really helped me control my blood sugar [glucose], but you won't believe how much weight I have lost.* Even more common is the second pattern of comments something like this: *Wow! I've lost so much weight. And by the way, my blood sugar control is much better too.*

The success that readers have had losing weight based on my earlier books has motivated me to write this book with the expectation of helping Americans live a longer, healthier life.

What I've learned from my passion for controlling my blood glucose is this very simple truth which has become the first principle of the Glucose Control Diet©: *If you control your blood glucose, you control your weight.*

To understand how to control your blood glucose and lose weight, you must first understand how your body *both* gains and loses weight.

You will learn that in the next chapter.

Chapter 2

How Our Bodies Gain
and Lose Weight

In this book, I am not just going to tell you what to eat to lose weight. I want you to *understand* the simple process of losing weight permanently.

I won't ask you to try to memorize what to eat and what not to eat. I won't ask you to measure grams or ounces of foods. I won't even ask you to count calories in your meals. None of those steps has worked for America. We've tried them all and we still get fatter.

What I will do is ask you to start your journey to a slimmer, healthier self by reading this chapter carefully. By the time you finish this chapter, you will understand, in everyday language, your body's process of losing weight and gaining weight.

By the time you finish *this book*, you will also know which groups of foods and which foods within those groups to eat to lose weight and which foods to avoid and why. You will also know which foods to combine and which not to combine to lose weight.

When you understand what to eat to lose weight and avoid ever gaining it back, you will be on your way to a slimmer, healthier life.

The Role of Food and the Role of Exercise in Gaining and Losing Weight

Weight loss and weight gain are determined by what we put into our bodies and how we burn what we put in. Both are important *but what we put into our body for energy and storage has a much greater impact on weight gain or weight loss than how we burn that food.*

You can't lose weight by eating badly and exercising rigorously. To say it another way, "You can't lose weight by trying to outwork bad eating habits."

But you can lose weight by eating correctly without much exercise. I do not recommend doing that because there are so many cardiovascular and general health benefits in aerobic exercise whether walking, running, biking, or just moving more in your daily activity.

For most adults—who are not training for aerobic competitions or who don't have physically demanding jobs—what we put into our bodies for energy has about 80% of the impact on weight and how we burn that energy has about 20% of the impact on weight. This is commonly accepted wisdom by medical professionals and their unconventional bedfellows, bodybuilders.

I have also found this to be true myself by measuring my blood glucose after good meals, after bad meals, after no exercise, and after a lot of exercise.

Because what you eat has a greater impact on weight than exercise, this book is primarily about what we put into our bodies with a smaller part of the book dedicated to activity and exercise. This is by no means discounting the value of both aerobic and strength-building exercise. Both are good for general health, longevity, and a good quality of life.

If you don't change your activity level, the amount of glucose you cause to enter your bloodstream is the sole determiner of weight gain and weight loss. If you eat foods that create a lot of glucose in your bloodstream, you will get fatter. If you eat foods that create a small amount of glucose in your bloodstream, you will get thinner.

How Do I Know so Much About Glucose Control and Why Is that Important to You?

From the age of 20, when I was first diagnosed with type 1 diabetes, to my current age of 78, being aware of the glucose created by what I ate or drank was an essential part of my life. Although I have had diabetes for 58 years and counting, self-testing of blood glucose has been available for only about 40 years.

Because I am a Type 1 diabetic, my pancreas doesn't balance my blood glucose as it does in nondiabetics. I must continually measure and balance my blood glucose myself.

To master that balancing act and live the long, healthy life I have, I've embraced the challenge of avoiding both high and low blood glucose by testing my own blood for glucose five times a day in my earlier testing years, now more than 10 times a day. I estimate that I have given myself more than 85,000 blood glucose tests over the past 40 years since self-testing has become available.

I have tested multiple times after nearly every meal I have eaten and many times after snacks as well. I also measure before and after exercise so I can assess how the food is burned.

I have had to learn how to control my blood glucose to avoid the devastating consequences and the short, unhealthy life of a poorly controlled diabetic. My lean physique and exceptional health are the beneficial side effects of learning which foods will create high blood glucose and which foods will not.

In order to share this information on controlling blood glucose with the approximately 3 million Type 1 diabetics and the 30 million or more Type 2 diabetics, I've charted and graphed many of these tests and published them in two of the three books I've written about blood glucose control for diabetics.

What Should I Eat? to Solve Diabetes, Lose Weight, and Live Healthy and *Your Type 2 diabetes lifeline.*

The foods I have learned to eat to keep my blood glucose down and have taught Type 2 diabetics to eat to keep their blood glucose down, are *exactly* the foods all overweight people must eat to lose weight.

Now I want to share this information with those overweight or obese folks who would like to lose weight and also with those who are okay with their weight now but want to avoid the gradual weight gain that seems to come as Americans get older.

If you would like to lose weight in a healthy and permanent way, reading this book and applying this information will not only make your pounds melt away but will also improve your mobility, your quality of life, and the length of your healthy life.

—————

What I've Learned about Foods, Blood Glucose, and Weight Control.

As a well-known person in my home state of Alaska and as someone who has been open about living with Type 1 diabetes for most of my life, I often got requests to speak about living a full and healthy life with diabetes. Now, my speech requests have evolved to answering the question Alaskans and most Americans have about weight, "What Should I Eat to Lose Weight and Live a Longer, Healthier Life?"

Over the years, I've made presentations to medical associations, medical school classes, service clubs, diabetes events, high schools, universities, health fairs, clinics, and hospitals.

Controlling your blood glucose is the key to both controlling diabetes and losing weight. I've spent my life learning how to control my blood glucose to live a healthy life with Type 1 diabetes. Now I'm going to teach you how to control your blood glucose to lose weight.

Here's what I've learned over the past 40 years of testing about the relationship between glucose and weight gain.

At the end of each day, my insulin pump tells me how much insulin I've pumped in that day. If what I've eaten over a period of a week produces an amount of glucose in my bloodstream that requires me to give myself an average of 30 units or more of insulin a day, I will gain weight during that week.

If the food I eat over a week's time produces glucose in my bloodstream that requires me to give myself between 25 and 30 units of insulin a day for a week, I neither gain nor lose weight.

Now, getting to the important point; if the food I eat produces an amount of glucose in my bloodstream that only requires me to give myself 20 to 25 units of insulin a day for a week, I will lose weight.

What most people don't understand and what you will learn in this book is that blood glucose (sugar) is not created just by eating sweets. It's created by all food groups and all individual foods we eat or drink. Some foods create lots of glucose and some foods create very little glucose.

Two factors were critically important as I measured the impact of foods on my blood glucose. First, of course, was how much glucose the foods created, and second was how fast the glucose entered my bloodstream. You will later learn why these two factors, the size of the increase in glucose and the speed of the increase are important to weight loss.

Will the Size and Speed of the Blood Glucose Increases Be the Same for Everyone?

In general, yes. This is the very same reason that all weight-loss books can tell you to limit sweets. Sweets create lots of blood glucose for everybody and create it quickly. That adds weight to all people with the only variable being the existing size and weight of the people eating or drinking the food.

Because we are talking about blood glucose action by the same foods, the *speed* at which it enters the bloodstream as glucose will, for all practical purposes, be the same for all people; but the *size* of the increases in blood glucose from the same foods will vary based on the size and weight of the person eating.

I'm 6 feet 2 inches and weigh about 180 pounds. A person who weighs, say, 90 pounds more than I do would have a bigger volume of blood in his or her body. If they were to eat the same foods and *same portion size* I did, their blood sugar would not go up as much as mine would. Just as if you put a teaspoon of sugar in an 8 oz. glass of iced tea and your friend put the same amount of sugar in a 16 oz. glass of iced tea. Both people's iced tea would be impacted by the sugar at the same speed, but your friend's 16 oz. glass of iced tea would be only half as sweet as your 8 oz. glass.

The converse of this is true also. A smaller person—if he or she ate the same portion size of food that I did—would experience a greater rise of blood sugar but the speed it goes into the bloodstream would be the same.

That distinction, based on body size, is not critical to the message of this book. Even if you do not change the amount or portion size of the food you eat but follow my recommendations on *what* you should eat, you will create less glucose in your bloodstream and *you will lose weight and keep it off.*

If you lower your blood glucose your insulin demand will automatically go down. You will lose weight—and that is true for everyone. If you also lower your portion size you will create even less glucose in your bloodstream, and you will *lose even more weight.*

You now know that to reduce your insulin demand you must reduce the glucose (sugar) you put in your bloodstream.

So how do you lower your blood glucose and therefore your insulin demand?

The answer is this: You need to know which foods create more glucose and which foods create less glucose and which foods enter your bloodstream faster and which enter more slowly.

The above iced tea example says that both glasses would create the increase in sweetness at the same speed. It's true in that case because it's the same food (sugar) that you're putting in the iced tea, but not all foods enter your bloodstream as glucose at the same speed. Some foods create glucose that enters your bloodstream as glucose quickly and some foods enter your bloodstream as glucose slowly.

If you eat two foods that cause your blood glucose to increase by the same amount but one of those foods goes into your bloodstream faster, you will gain more weight from that fast-entering food than you will from the slow-entering food.

The reason that slow-entering food is better for weight-loss is simply that you will have more time to use the glucose that food creates. You will burn it as it more slowly enters your bloodstream *before* it gets stored as fat.

Conversely, you will be unlikely to burn all the glucose of the faster acting food before it gets stored as fat.

Before I introduce the four principles of the Glucose Control Diet©, you need to know, in everyday language, what happens when you eat or drink for nourishment. It's very important for you to understand how your body gains and loses weight.

What Happens in Our Bodies As We Eat or Drink for Nourishment?

First, I'm going to presume you don't have Type 2 diabetes as I explain what happens to nondiabetics as they eat. Then, because many of you who are reading this may already have—or will have— Type 2 diabetes, I'll explain what happens when a Type 2 diabetic, or borderline diabetic eats or drinks for nourishment.

The most common estimate is that about 80 percent of Type 2 diabetics are overweight or obese. When you combine that statistic with the Center for Disease Control's estimate that more than one-third of Americans are obese and another one-third are overweight but not classified as obese, you can understand why Type 2 diabetes may become a part of your future unless you embrace Glucose Control Eating©.

What Happens When a Person without Diabetes Eats for Energy and Nourishment?

When a nondiabetic eats food, *all* that food is converted to some amount of glucose. As you know, some foods convert to *large amounts* of glucose, other foods to *small amounts* of glucose. Some foods enter the bloodstream as glucose quickly. Other foods enter the bloodstream as glucose more slowly.

When glucose starts entering the bloodstream it triggers a rise in blood glucose (sugar). As the blood glucose begins to rise, a signal is sent to the pancreas to start producing insulin, which is the hormone that allows the glucose that goes into the bloodstream to be absorbed through walls of the bloodstream into the body's cells for energy and storage. In a nondiabetic, the pancreas obliges and produces just the right amount of insulin.

That insulin also allows the excess glucose that is not used for energy or stored in the liver, to be stored around the body as fat. That's an important point to remember. If you eat foods—or drinks— that create more glucose than is necessary for your immediate energy needs, that glucose will automatically be stored, first in the liver where it's called glycogen, then as body fat stored in all the places you don't want it stored.

When your pancreas has produced sufficient insulin to allow the body to use the glucose in your bloodstream and store the excess glucose in your liver, then the pancreas stops sending any more insulin to the bloodstream and the blood sugar stabilizes at a normal* level.

Think of it this way. For a nondiabetic, eating is like heating a house in the winter using a thermostat. When the house gets too cold, the

---

AUTHOR'S NOTE:

Normal level is generally considered to be between 75 and 105 mg/dl (that's milligrams of sugar (glucose) per deciliter of blood). You don't need to remember the "milligrams per deciliter" part but you do need to know the term, blood glucose ,and what the normal, healthy level is.

thermostat sends a message to the furnace that says, "Turn on the heat." When the furnace brings the heat up to the set (normal) temperature, the thermostat sends the signal to stop sending up heat.

That's the way things are supposed to work. But what if the pancreas has been overworked because of bad eating habits or a sedentary life and can't produce enough insulin? That's the challenge Type 2 diabetics have, and borderline, or pre-diabetics, will have if they don't take corrective or preventative action.

Now, What Happens When a Borderline Diabetic or Type 2 Diabetic Eats for Energy and Nourishment?

The process for a Type 2 diabetic is the same as for a nondiabetic—up to a point.

When a borderline or Type 2 diabetic eats food, *all* that food is converted into some amount of glucose exactly as it is with a nondiabetic. Some foods create *large amounts* of glucose, other foods *small amounts* of glucose just as in a nondiabetic. Some foods enter the bloodstream as glucose quickly. Other foods enter the bloodstream as glucose more slowly just as in a nondiabetic.

When glucose starts entering the bloodstream, a signal is sent to the pancreas to start producing insulin. This insulin allows the glucose going into the bloodstream to be absorbed through walls of the bloodstream into the body's cells for energy and storage; just as it does for a nondiabetic.

Here is where things change. In a Type 2 diabetic, the pancreas says, *"I've been working too hard trying to produce the insulin needed for all the glucose you've been creating. I am tired and I can't produce all the insulin you need. But I will produce what I can and hope it helps."* Implicit in this message is if the borderline or Type 2 diabetic will reduce the amount of glucose in the bloodstream, it will reduce the demand for insulin and the pancreas will be able to produce sufficient insulin to meet that demand.

Also, putting less glucose in the bloodstream will reduce the workload on the overworked pancreas of the borderline or Type 2 diabetic. That means you are giving your pancreas a rest and a chance to regenerate its insulin-producing capability.

If you do not change your diet and put less glucose in your bloodstream, your blood glucose will be constantly above normal. It is that higher-than-normal blood glucose that causes multiple health complications: circulatory problems, kidney failure, vision impairment or blindness, amputations of feet and legs, heart problems, and strokes.

By lowering and controlling your blood glucose, you can avoid the multiple complications of consistently high blood sugars.

If you are a borderline diabetic, The Glucose Control Diet™ will save you from getting Type 2 diabetes. If you already have Type 2 diabetes, you can—as many of the readers of my book, *Your Type 2 Diabetes Lifeline,* already have—reverse it and become nondiabetic.

The best action *Type 2 diabetics, pre-diabetics, or borderline diabetics* can take to avoid diabetic complications and eliminate the need to take medications or injections is to first lower your blood sugars. When you change your eating patterns to lower your blood sugar, your weight will start coming off. When those eating patterns become habits your weight will stay off. The result will be a healthier and longer life.

For those of you who already have Type 2 diabetes or are pre-diabetic or borderline diabetic, I recommend my book **Your Type 2 Diabetes Lifeline**. It is simple, clear, and filled with good information to help folks lose weight, live healthier, and avoid or banish Type 2 diabetes.

Chapter 3

The Five Principles of Weight Loss in Glucose Control Eating©

Introduction to the Principles of Weight Loss in the Glucose Control Diet

These five weight-loss principles are the foundation of Glucose Control Eating©. They will be explored, explained, and illustrated throughout the book. As you begin your journey to reach a healthy weight, to maintain that weight, and to feel better for the rest of your life, these five principles will guide you in that journey.

The First Principle of Weight Loss in Glucose Control Eating©

If You Control Your Blood Glucose, You Control Your Weight.
In this chapter I explain why glucose is your weight-loss stop-and-go light. As you now know, the amount of glucose you put into your bloodstream and the speed of that glucose entering your bloodstream determines your weight gain or weight loss. If you put too much glucose in your bloodstream, your weight loss stops. Put less glucose in your bloodstream and your weight loss continues. In future chapters, you will learn which foods create less glucose and which foods create more glucose. That information will be your weight-loss road map.

The Second Principle of Weight Loss in Glucose Control Eating©

All Foods We Eat: Proteins, Fats, and Carbohydrates Put Some Amount of Glucose into Our Bloodstreams.
It is not just sweets that create glucose in your bloodstream. All foods do. Some foods and drinks create a lot of glucose and some create a small amount of glucose.

Since the amount of glucose created by the foods you eat—or drink—will determine your weight loss, it is important that you know which categories of foods create less glucose and which categories create more glucose. You need that information to lose weight easily and keep it off permanently. In upcoming chapters, you will learn which food categories and which individual foods are your weight-loss friends and which are not.

The Third Principle of Weight Loss in Glucose Control Eating©

Carbohydrates cannot be considered as a single food group for weight loss. In Glucose Control Eating©, carbohydrates (carbs) are divided into four subgroups based on their impact on weight.
From elementary school through high school and college, we have been taught the *three food groups*: proteins, fats, and carbohydrates. This is one of the biggest problems for people trying to lose weight, because carbohydrates are too broad a group for anyone to say, eat fewer carbs to lose weight.

In the standard way of looking at food groups, the best way of describing a carbohydrate is, *if it is not a protein or fat, it is a carbohydrate*. Most proteins are similar in their impact on blood sugars and therefore on weight. Most fats are similar in that regard also. But carbohydrates? They are all over the board in terms of impact on blood glucose and weight.

Based on what I learned from my more than 40 years of blood glucose testing, I have divided carbohydrates into four distinct groups based on how much and how fast they impact blood glucose. Here are the four sub-groups of carbs: *sweet carbs, starchy carbs, fruit carbs, and vegetable (veggie) carbs.*

Throughout this book you will learn which of these sub-groups of carbs you should eat more of and which you should eat less of.

The Fourth Principle of Weight Loss in Glucose Control Eating©

Foods that enter your bloodstream more slowly contribute to more weight loss than foods that enter your bloodstream faster.
Now that you know that the amount of glucose foods create is a major determiner of weight gain and weight loss, I'm going to complicate it a bit by adding another factor: *how fast foods enter your bloodstream as glucose is also an important weight loss issue.*

The glucose that enters your bloodstream quickly from the foods you eat is more likely to be stored as fat before you can use it. Foods that create glucose in your bloodstream slowly give your body more time to burn that glucose before it is stored as fat.

Later in this book, you will read and see why this is such an important factor and which foods enter your bloodstream as glucose slowly and which do not.

The Fifth Principle of Weight Loss in Glucose Control Eating©

When foods are combined with other foods, the combined foods have a different impact on your blood glucose and weight than if the foods were eaten separately.
To my knowledge, this principle of combined foods has never been published and quite possibly never been researched.

Later in this book, you will see graphs showing which combinations of foods raise your blood glucose more and which combinations raise your blood glucose less.

It's obvious from these five principles of Glucose Control Eating©, that the key to losing weight is to understand how much and how fast different foods and combinations of foods will raise your blood glucose.

That may seem like a daunting task, but because I categorize foods by their impact on blood glucose and illustrate this in graphs, you will be surprised at how easy it will be for you to learn and remember which food groups and foods will cause you to gain weight and which will cause you to lose weight. With this knowledge, you will be surprised at how easily the pounds and inches will disappear from the start with The Glucose Control Eating©.

More Detail on the Five Principles of Weight-Loss with the Glucose Control Diet©

Now that you've been introduced to the five principles Glucose Control Eating©, here's a little more detail on each of the principles. Throughout this book, I will be applying these three principles to various foods and combinations of foods.

Principle I
If you control your blood glucose, you control your weight

Put more glucose into your bloodstream, and you will gain weight. Put less glucose into your bloodstream, and you will lose weight. This a fact that is not disputed by medical doctors or medical researchers.

The focus of this book is to not only tell you which foods create less glucose but also to show you graphically which foods create less glucose.

You may forget some of the foods that will accelerate your weight loss, but you will easily conjure up the image of the graphs showing weight gain or loss and remember the foods that way.

Doctors often tell overweight patients who have Type 2 diabetes, if they want to lower their blood glucose (blood sugar), they *should* lose weight. That is not incorrect, but I tell people the converse of that: if you lower your blood glucose, you *will* lose weight.

As I share this with doctors in the many speeches I have given with members of medical communities in attendance, I see many positive nods of heads as if to say, "Hmm, that makes sense." When I share this statement with doctors in personal conversations, I hear many say they will change the order of their advice.

But Isn't Insulin the Fat Traffic Light?

Insulin is often called "nature's fat traffic light" because the more insulin your body produces the more weight you will gain. The less insulin your body produces the more weight you will lose. Then which is it that causes weight gain or loss? Is it insulin or is it glucose?

Insulin allows the glucose in your bloodstream to get into your cells to be used for energy and storage. The pancreas produces insulin in response to the glucose in your bloodstream. Put more glucose in your bloodstream in your bloodstream and your pancreas produces more insulin; put less glucose in your bloodstream and your pancreas produces less insulin.

The next time you read or hear that too much *insulin* is the cause of weight gain remember that insulin is just the responder. Too much glucose in your bloodstream is what triggers more insulin and creates more weight.

As you continue reading this book and understand the graphs, you will remember this principle. Within just a few *days* after finishing this book and applying what you have learned, you will be a believer in Glucose Control Eating© because your weight loss will have already started.

You are now aware that putting too much glucose in your bloodstream will cause you to gain weight and putting smaller amounts of glucose in your bloodstream will cause you to lose weight. The logical question for you to ask is, "What should I eat to reduce the amount of glucose I put in my bloodstream?"

This brings us to the second principle of weight loss with the Glucose Control Diet.

Principle 2

All foods we eat—proteins, fats, and carbohydrates, turn into some amount of glucose in our bloodstreams.

Glucose in your bloodstream does not come just from eating sweets. Glucose comes from all foods we eat. Some foods will turn into a lot of glucose and other foods will turn into just a little glucose.

Proteins like seafood and meat convert to glucose in your blood, but convert to small amounts of glucose.

Fats also convert to small amounts of glucose in your blood and also go in very slowly.

Some carbohydrates convert to a lot of glucose in your bloodstream while other carbohydrates contribute little glucose to your bloodstream. Still other carbohydrates are somewhere in between.

Because carbs vary so much in their impact on blood glucose and therefore on weight, learning which is which is your key to lower blood glucose, weight loss, and a healthier life.

Principle 3
Carbohydrates cannot be considered as a single food group for weight loss. In Glucose Control Eating©, carbohydrates (carbs) are divided into four sub-groups based on their impact on weight.

Most people can name proteins—meats, fish, some vegetables. And most people have some grasp of natural fats—bacon, olive oil, butter, fatty meats, and fatty fish. But ask an American to name carbohydrates and you will get an uncertain look and some guesses.

For example, cauliflower is a carbohydrate and so is a bagel. Spaghetti's a carbohydrate and so is an apple. Bread is a carbohydrate and so is broccoli. Cereal is a carbohydrate and so is cabbage. Pastas are carbohydrates and so is a grapefruit. So how can you possibly talk about carbohydrates in general because they are such a broad category and so different in their impact on blood glucose and weight?

No wonder people are confused when they are told to "eat fewer carbs." Does that mean eat less broccoli, fewer apples, less corn?

To clarify this carb and weight-loss confusion, I use a new and better way of grouping foods based on how much and how fast different foods raise blood glucose and contribute to weight.

The next three chapters will provide the information on food groups to help you understand what to eat and what not to eat—or more accurately, which foods to eat more of and which foods to eat less of to lose weight.

Here's an introduction to the six food groups that will help clarify the role of carbohydrates in weight loss in the glucose control diet©. Those food groups are four sub-groups of carbohydrates plus protein and fat.

1. *Sweet carbohydrates* like sugared soft drinks, candy, doughnuts, cakes, pies, and many other sugared desserts, of course, turn into a lot of glucose and enter your bloodstream quickly.

2. *Starchy carbohydrates* like bread, bagels, spaghetti, pasta, potatoes, and rice also turn into a lot of glucose and enter your bloodstream quickly.

3. *Fruit Carbohydrates* put glucose in your bloodstream but in general not as much glucose as sweet or starchy carbs and enter your bloodstream a little more slowly than sweet or starchy carbs. You will learn later in this book which fruits do contribute to significant weight gain and which fruits do not.

4. *Vegetable Carbohydrates* also create some glucose in your bloodstream, but less than fruits and much less than sweet and starchy carbs. And as an additional benefit, vegetables' conversion to glucose is slow, which gives you a chance to burn the small amount of glucose they create before it's stored in your liver as glycogen and on your body as fat. Going in slowly also means you will not be hungry again as quickly as you would be with sweet or starchy carbs.

5. *Proteins* also create way less glucose than sweet and starchy carbs, less than fruits, and slightly less than most vegetables. Proteins are also slow to convert to glucose, which means it will have a longer time to be burned before they are stored as body fat. Proteins will also postpone any feelings of hunger longer than sweet or starchy carbs.

6. Finally, *fats* also create some glucose but go into your bloodstream more slowly than all other food groups. This slowness is good because even with a minimal amount of activity you can burn most of it before it gets stored as body fat. Fat will also delay, for about three to five hours, any feeling of hunger.

In conclusion, lock this into your memory: *Everything you eat creates blood glucose. Eat foods that put less glucose into your bloodstream, you will lose weight. Eat foods that put more glucose in your bloodstream, you will gain weight. How do you know which foods to eat to lose weight? This book will show you.*

Principle 4
Foods that enter your bloodstream more slowly contribute more to weight loss than foods that enter your bloodstream faster.
Both the amount of increase and the speed of increase of blood glucose have a big impact on weight gain.

Foods that go into your bloodstream slowly are good for two reasons. They give you a chance to burn the glucose created before it is stored as body fat *and* they postpone the feelings of hunger for much longer that fast-entering foods.

The foods that go into your bloodstream too fast are likely to be stored as body fat before you can burn the glucose they create. After eating those foods, you will also be hungry within a couple of hours and tempted to snack or eat again.

This slowness of conversion to glucose is another subject that, to the best of my knowledge, has never before been published in any book, magazine, or journal.

The final principle is another one that I have never seen discussed before: how foods act in combinations.

Principle 5
When foods are combined with other foods, the combined foods have a different impact on your weight than if the foods were eaten separately.
Fat is a friend of weight loss under certain conditions. Fats can be eaten freely in combination with some foods with little impact on weight but in combinations with other foods is a big contributor to weight gain.

The impact of fats has been the biggest revelation to me over my years of testing. It took me over two decades and thousands of blood tests to realize that fat alone has minimal impact on my blood glucose and almost no impact on weight gain, provided it is combined with protein or vegetables.

But if fat is combined in a meal with starchy carbs or followed by a dessert of sweet carbs, it is a big contributor to weight gain.

Fat alone or with vegetables or protein is not the villain it is made out to be. I know this is going to be a hard paradigm shift for Americans, because for years we have read over and over about losing weight with low-fat diets. We have read about low-fat this and low-fat that. Who argued? It seemed so reasonable. If you don't want to get fat, don't eat fat. Right? No. Wrong.

Fat is a very stable molecule and hard to break down. It is the slowest of all foods to convert to glucose. Because it is so slow to convert to glucose, you will have plenty of time to burn that glucose before it is stored. Fat will also keep you from getting hungry for a much longer time than sweet carbs or starchy carbs.

Fats, if eaten alone or with vegetables or proteins, are contributors to increased HDL (good cholesterol). Much more on this later in this book. As you will see in upcoming chapters, many researchers are now promoting fat as a healthy part of eating.

Chapter 4

The Six Food Groups of Glucose Control Eating©

The New and Better Way of Grouping Foods for Weight Loss Based on *How Much* and *How Fast* Foods Will Raise Blood Glucose and Add Weight

This new look at food groups will help you understand what to eat and what not to eat—or more accurately which foods to eat more of and which foods to eat less of to lose weight.

This chapter provides a new look at food groups that will clarify what foods to eat to make your pounds disappear and never return.

I first introduced this concept of six food groups based on their impact on glucose in my book, *Your Type 2 Diabetes Lifeline*, to help Type 2 diabetics lower their blood glucose and reverse Type 2 diabetes. The feedback I got from readers of that book was positive about their success in lowering their blood sugars, but it was unexpectedly exuberant about the side effect of weight loss they all experienced.

As you are introduced to this new way of grouping foods based on weight loss, remember **The Second Principle of Glucose Control Eating©**.

All foods we eat—proteins, fats, and carbohydrates, turn into some amount of glucose in our bloodstreams.

The Six Food Groups You Need to Understand

Here are the new six discrete groups of foods you need to understand to lower your blood glucose, lose weight, and live healthier:

Sweet carbohydrates

Starchy carbohydrates

Fruit carbohydrates

Vegetable (veggie) Carbohydrates

Proteins

Fats

Each of these categories of foods plays a different role in blood glucose control and weight gain or loss.

Once you understand how each category of food impacts your blood glucose and weight control, improving your health and losing weight will be surprisingly easy.

The beauty of this categorization is you don't have to try to memorize how hundreds—or thousands—of foods impact your blood sugar and weight; you just need to understand how these six categories of foods impact your blood sugar and weight.

Now let's look in more detail at these categories.

Understand the Six Food Groups of Glucose Control Eating©

Sweet Carbohydrates—The Enemy We Know

Sweet carbs are made up of simple molecules—mostly lone molecules or maybe two stuck together. They are *easily dissolved and quick to enter your bloodstream*. You will see in the graphs they are the quickest of the food categories to enter your bloodstream and will cause the greatest rise in your blood glucose. They also get out of your bloodstream quickly and you will be hungry again more quickly than you will be with other foods. This is nothing new, but sweets are a big problem for anyone who wants to lose weight.

Remember that a rise in blood glucose means more insulin demand, which means more weight gain. In the next chapter, you will see graphs of how fast and how much this group will raise your blood sugar compared to other groups. Those visuals will help you lock into your mind the impact of sweets on weight gain.

Examples of Sweet Carbohydrates
Here are examples of foods included in this category:

sugared soft drinks	sorbets
cakes	chocolates
pies	caramels
donuts	a broad selection of desserts
sweet rolls	and of course, almost all candies
ice cream, sherbets, and	

Some of these foods also have starchy carbs and fat in them. Later you will learn that a combination of sweet carbs and fat will cause big rises in blood glucose.

We all know by now that too much sugar is the villain, right? Then what about all the *sugar-free* candies? Are they okay? They taste just like regular candy. What a good find. Now I can eat all the candy I want. Right? No. Wrong!

Look closely at the label. You'll see that many of those items are sweetened with high-fructose corn syrup or with other sweeteners not much different from cane sugar except that they are more concentrated, and most make you even fatter than cane sugar. Do not think you are doing yourself a favor by eating sugar-free candy. In terms of impact on blood sugar and weight, sugar-free candies often have greater impact than candy sweetened with cane sugar.

Both regular candy and sugar-free candy are items you need to start minimizing dramatically. This is, of course, not new information, but if you do the other things I propose and still eat candy, you are not going to make the progress you want.

How about desserts? Take heart. In the next few chapters on actions to control blood glucose and lose weight, I am not going to talk about cutting out all desserts all the time. But I will be talking about dramatically minimizing both the frequency and the quantity of sweet desserts.

Okay. No big surprise about sweet carbs being bad but once you see the graphs, you'll see how bad they really are for weight loss.

The next category is one that will surprise quite a few people.

Starchy Carbohydrates—The Enemy Many of Us Don't Know

Starchy carbs have a slightly more complex molecular structure than sweet carbohydrates. Their molecules are stuck together in larger strings or branching chains which are slightly harder to break apart and are just a little bit slower to enter your bloodstream than sweets. However, you will see in the graphs that they cause a rise in your blood glucose similar to that of sweet carbs.

Examples of Starchy Carbohydrates

Here are some examples of foods included in this category:

waffles

pancakes

dry breakfast cereals
(sweetened or not)

white bread of all kinds

multi-grain breads
*whole grain is better
than multi-grain*

rolls

hamburger and hot dog buns

muffins

bagels

tortillas

tortilla chips

potato chips

crackers

spaghetti

lasagna

pasta

white rice

brown rice
*brown rice is slightly better
than white rice*

Fruit Carbohydrates—the Good Fruits for Weight Loss and the Not-So-Good

This category has a bit of variation in how fast and how much different fruits will increase blood sugar. Some fruit carbs act relatively slowly and cause moderate increases in blood sugar and weight gain, and some enter the bloodstream more quickly and will cause a bigger increase in blood glucose and weight gain. This requires some distinction to be made within the category.

While fruits are not a free ride in terms of blood glucose and weight, many fruits do contain a variety of vitamins, minerals, and fiber which are important to good health. You will see from the graphs that some fruits will raise your blood sugar quickly and contribute significantly to weight gain and some will have a small impact on blood glucose and weight gain.

Examples of Fruit Carbohydrates
Many fruits will raise your blood glucose quickly and need to be moderated. The fruits in this category are the following:

pineapples	pears
bananas	grapes
cherries peaches	strawberries

Other fruits raise blood glucose more slowly and can be eaten more freely. The fruits in this category are the following:

cantaloupe	raspberries
blueberries	grapefruit
blackberries	and—surprisingly—oranges

I do not mean to imply that you can't eat fruits if you want to lose weight, but they are not a free ride with regard to blood glucose and weight. Eat more of the fruits on the second list and less of the fruits on the first list.

How about fruit juices?

I've found that many fruit juices are problematic because they cause very fast and very big blood glucose increases. In many cases a small glass of *apple* juice or *orange* juice for breakfast will raise my blood glucose more than all the rest of my breakfast combined. And it gets into my bloodstream much faster than I can generally use it, so gets stored first in my liver then in and around my body as fat.

An Associated Press article in the December 11, 2011 edition of the *Honolulu Star* supports what I learned decades ago. The headline states, "Apple juice is far from nutritious, experts say." The article continues "…nutrition experts say apple juice's real danger is to waistlines and children's teeth. Apple juice has few natural nutrients, lots of calories, and in some cases, more sugar than soda. It trains a child to like very sweet things, displaces better beverages and foods, and adds to the obesity problem."

Apple juice, orange juice, cranberry juice, and pineapple juice all make my blood glucose rise substantially and quickly and require me to take far more insulin and therefore contributes far more to my weight than the fruits themselves do. V-8 and grapefruit juices do not raise my blood sugar as much and are better choices.

If you are going to drink any of the above fruit juices, dilute them to about 25 percent juice with about 75 percent water or sparkling mineral water. In other words, one part juice to three parts club soda or a sparkling water such as Pellegrino or Perrier. You will soon get accustomed to the less sweet taste of diluted juices.

For anyone trying to lower blood glucose and lose weight, the best juice to drink by far as you will see in the next chapter is V-8 juice. I have found that V-8 juice mixed with lemon- or lime-flavored sparkling water makes a very refreshing drink during the day and—with or without a few spices—makes a nice, nonalcoholic cocktail in the evening.

I've also found that mixing a half cup of V-8 juice with a half cup of whole milk heated in a microwave for 90 seconds makes an easy, good-tasting, healthy version of tomato-like soup without all the sugar that most tomato soups have.

For those looking for a lower-sodium drink, V-8 also has a low-sodium version.

Veggie Carbohydrates—A Great Friend of Weight Loss

Veggie carbs have a more complex molecular structure than sweet or starchy carbohydrates. You'll see in the graphs they are much *slower* to enter your bloodstream than either sweet or starchy carbs and slightly slower than most fruit carbs. Almost all veggie carbohydrates will also raise your blood glucose less than sweet carbs, starchy carbs, or fruit carbs.

Because vegetables will cause a very small and very slow increase in blood glucose, you will burn most of that small amount of glucose created by veggie carbs before it gets stored in your liver as glycogen or around your body as fat.

Examples of Veggie Carbohydrates

These are the foods your mom told you to eat. She was right. They include most vegetables including but not limited to the following:

asparagus	lettuce
broccoli	peppers
tomatoes	mushrooms
cauliflower	peas
Brussels sprouts	beans
artichokes	beets
spinach	sauerkraut
cabbage	salad greens.

You can eat as much as you want of these vegetables and—as you will see later—you can use butter freely with them with little or no impact on your blood glucose or weight.

Three vegetables that do cause slightly higher and faster increases than the other vegetables are ***corn, potatoes, and carrots***. These three foods have much more nutritional benefit than sweet or starchy carbs. While you shouldn't eat them with abandon, just moderate the portions. Don't eliminate them.

In the next few chapters, you will see that I speak often of maximizing protein, fat, and veggie carbohydrates, moderating fruit carbs, minimizing starchy carbs, and eliminating or cutting way back on sweet carbohydrates.

Now let's look at protein.

Protein—A Good Friend of Weight Loss That Has Gone in and out of Favor over the Years.

The molecular structure of protein is more complex than the previous four food categories and therefore slower to enter your bloodstream as glucose than sweet carbs, starchy carbs, and fruit carbs and about the same as or slightly slower than most veggie carbs. As with veggie carbs, the rise in your blood sugar caused by proteins will be neither fast nor significant.

Protein has gone in and out of favor many times in the past 60 years but from the past 35 years of my blood sugar testing, I've learned that protein has very little effect on my blood glucose and a very noticeably positive effect on my muscle growth when I match protein with modest strength training.

Because protein will cause neither a quick nor a significant rise in blood glucose, I freely eat protein. That slow insignificant rise in blood glucose means—like vegetables—not only will these foods be burned before they are stored but also, they will require your body to burn existing glycogen from your liver and then burn fat stored around your body.

Protein is the other food group—along with vegetables—that you can eat with butter or fat-based sauces with little impact on weight except to lose it. Protein with vegetables and butter or fat-based sauces (with no flour or sugar added) are excellent meals to meet your weight-loss goals.

Examples of Protein

Here are examples of protein you can eat often and freely to meet your weight-loss goals as long as they are not combined with starchy or sweet carbs.

Fish and Seafood

salmon	shrimp
halibut	scallops
crab	catfish
cod	sunfish
pollock	pike
lobster	tuna
trout	

Poultry

chicken	Cornish game hen
turkey	*all okay to eat with the skin but not with breading*
eggs	

Eggs are a mixture of protein and fat that you can eat freely, and will have little impact on your blood glucose, weight, or cholesterol (more on this later).

Meat

steak	mutton
prime rib	rack-of-lamb
ham	lamb chops
pork	corned beef
bacon	

(As an aside, I personally don't eat veal because of the distressing way calves are confined for their whole lives to improve the taste and tenderness of veal).

You do *not* have to limit your meats to only lean meat as you will often read. That statement is a holdover from the terribly inaccurate

Food Pyramid that contributed to the obesity and Type 2 diabetes epidemics. As you study the graphs, you'll learn that you can *freely eat* meat marbled with fat and chicken and turkey *with* the skin.

Later in this chapter and in the next two chapters you'll see my defense of fat and read about how medical opinions about dietary fat are evolving.

Although the skin on poultry and the fat on meat are not a problem, *breading* (a starchy carb) on these foods is a problem if you are trying to lower your blood glucose and lose weight.

My core protein food is wild salmon (not farmed salmon). I eat it two or three times a week in the summer and fall but less frequently in the winter and spring.

It's an almost perfect food with minimal impact on blood sugar. Because it goes in so slowly it gets burned before it can be stored as fat on your body. It's very high in protein and high in omega-3 fatty acids, which my secondary research indicates is an exceptionally good fat. Salmon is also a good source of vitamin D. All that, and it tastes great too…providing you don't overcook it.

Fats

Not many foods are all or even predominantly fat, but here are a few of the foods that I include in the fat category:

butter	mayonnaise
olive oil	avocados
nuts	many salad dressings
peanut butter	

Proteins that are high in fat

These are foods that you can eat freely with little impact on blood sugar and weight—providing you follow my rules on when to eat fat and what not to combine it with.

eggs (with the yolk)	salmon
pork	rib-eye steaks
bacon	hamburger
prime rib	mutton
spareribs	

Because protein and fat are often present in the same foods, it is difficult to test just fat but more practical to test protein and fat together. Butter and olive oil are exceptions and can be tested with or without protein.

I make a distinction between "natural fats" and processed fats. I'm not personally knowledgeable in the category of processed fats because I do not knowingly eat them and consequently have not tested them. But I am very apprehensive about the taste enhancers and chemicals added during the processing.

Examples of this type of fats you should avoid are the following:

margarine	processed sandwich meats
fake butters	precooked frozen lunches and
hot dogs	dinners.

Evolving Medical Opinions on Fat

Some doctors and researchers who I will refer to later are leading the charge on this issue of fat not being your enemy, but it took more than 30 years for the federal bureaucracy to finally—and very quietly—admit the food pyramid was wrong and make a change to what they call "My Plate" which is better, but still not great for weight loss.

Fats Enter Your Bloodstream Very Slowly

Because the molecular structure of fat is complex and stable, it is slow to break down and enter your bloodstream as glucose. Fat with seafood and vegetables is a great, tasty, healthy combination of food for weight loss.

Let me say this again. *Fat has little impact on your blood sugar or on weight gain unless—as you will learn later—it's combined with starchy carbs in the same meal or with sweet carbs in that meal or in a dessert.*

Because this approach to fat is so different from what we have been taught for so many years, I refer to other researchers' opinions on fat in chapter 6.

Now that I've told you about the six food groups categorized by their influence on weight, I'm going to help you visually lock those groups into your mind with the graphs in the following chapter. You'll also be able to visualize how individual foods within those groups will influence body fat gain or body fat loss.

Chapter 5

The Glucose Control Graphs that Will Change Your Life

Graphs of Groups of Foods and Individual Foods That Are Your Key to Weight-loss Success

More than 40 Years of Testing Foods' Impact on Blood Glucose and Weight

It's taken me more than 40 years, and more than 85,000 blood glucose tests, to learn what you will learn from these graphs in about 40 minutes. They are your key to losing weight and maintaining that healthier weight for the rest of your life.

Before Self-testing Was Available

Though I've had Type 1 diabetes for 58 years and counting, self-testing has been available for only about 40 years. In the years before self-testing, the only way I could get a blood glucose measurement was to set an appointment with my doctor, who would give me a lab request. I then had to go to a lab to have a blood sample taken from a vein in my arm. The local lab would send it out to an analytical lab and get the result back in three days. The local lab would then call my doctor, who had a staff person call me and tell me what my blood sugar had been **three or four days** prior. Because of that cumbersome process, I had my blood sugar tested only three or four times a year during my first 16 or so years with diabetes.

After Self-Testing

Now I self-test when I wake up each morning, before and after most meals, often between meals, and twice before I go to bed each night—about an hour apart. I also test before and after physical activities and any other time I think my blood glucose needs adjusting. As a result of all these tests I've learned how hundreds—perhaps thousands—of different foods and combinations of foods impact my blood sugar and weight. I've learned not only how *much* different foods raise my blood but also how *fast* those foods raise my blood sugar.

What I Can't Measure

This is a good time to state that I can't make any judgments from my empirical testing of foods regarding their content of vitamins, minerals, or other ingredients that don't relate to blood sugar.

What I Can Measure

What I can and do measure, of course, is blood glucose, which is the determining factor in your weight. It is also a huge factor in your general health. High blood sugars, over time, will negatively affect your circulation, your pancreas, your kidneys, your liver, your heart, your feet, your vison, and your longevity.

Improving your blood glucose control will dramatically improve your health and your life expectancy,

Who will Benefit from This Information?

This information is written primarily for the more than two thirds of American adults who the Center for Disease Control says are overweight or obese and would like to lose weight. It is also critical for anyone with Type 2 diabetes pre-diabetes, or borderline diabetes. It will also be beneficial to all those who are happy with their current weight and who would just like to live a longer, healthier life without gaining weight.

The Purpose of the Graphs

The purpose of the graphs I present in this chapter is to provide visual representations of foods and combinations of foods to eat to lose weight and avoid gaining it back. These graphs will make it easier for the readers to *visualize and remember* which food groups—and foods within the groups—will add weight and which food groups and foods will not.

As you now know, since I'm a Type 1 diabetic, my body produces no insulin at all but whatever foods or combinations of foods I eat are converted to glucose in my blood just as they are for everyone, diabetic or not. But if I don't give myself a shot of insulin when I eat that food, my blood glucose will just keep on rising until I do give myself a shot.

Eating foods and not giving myself any insulin for 90 minutes is precisely how I can measure the blood glucose impact and therefore weight gain impact of individual foods and combinations of foods.

The graphs are a result of specific tests of blood glucose and weight gain impact of multiple foods and combinations of foods in the six food groups I use for the Glucose Control Diet™.

The graphs will clearly show what foods you should *minimize* to avoid weight gain and what foods you can *maximize*—with little rise in blood glucose—to promote weight loss. The results will surprise you …and change your life.

My Methodology for Testing

For the purposes of developing the graphs in this book I have conducted tests with a specific and consistent protocol.

I first made sure my blood glucose was stable. To assure stability, most of my tests were done in the morning when I hadn't eaten anything for at least 10 hours. To confirm that stability, I tested two or three times before I ate or drank the foods or drinks to be tested.

If my blood glucose was stable, I consumed the test foods or drinks. The next step was to set my smart-phone to alert me every 10 minutes for 90 minutes.

I made a special effort to keep my activity constant during the tests so the results would not be skewed by varying my activity. I usually read three newspapers on my iPad, read my emails, or planned my day during the 90 minutes of the tests.

During the tests, I was nine steps away from the counter upon which my testers and the charts were placed. That meant 18 steps back and forth every ten minutes for each test. Counting duplicate tests to confirm results, on average I stuck my fingers and tested my blood glucose about 12 to 15 times within a given test period.

At the end of 90 minutes and after all the results were recorded, I took an appropriate shot of insulin which—in a little more than an hour—brought my blood glucose back to a normal range.

Those 90 minutes tell a dramatic, visual story. They tell a story that can improve the lives of millions of Americans, a story that can help millions of people lose weight and prevent millions from ever getting Type 2 diabetes.

Indexing the Tests

The final point I need to make in describing my methodology is that at whatever stable point my blood was when I started, I indexed it to 100. What that means is if I established that my starting blood sugar was say 112 and stable, then my index was minus 12. That means I subtracted 12 points from my starting level and 12 points from every measurement for the full 90 minutes. And if for example my starting point was 84, I added 16 points to my starting level and 16 to each test for the full 90 minutes. That process gives every test the same starting point of 100 and will show accurate slopes, peaks, and areas that can be easily compared.

The findings are dramatic and may be different from what you've read or been told about food. The conclusions will provide you the information to change your eating lifestyle, your health, and your enjoyment of life. It's not about a short-term diet but rather about eating in a healthy way that you will enjoy for the rest of your life—eating *smaller* portions of the foods that maximize your blood sugars and contribute to weight gain and eating *larger* portions of the foods that have minimal effect on blood sugars and which will contribute to weight loss.

Will the foods I've Graphed Have the Same Impact on Everyone Else as They Have Had on Me?

The answer is, in general, yes. In terms of speed of entry into the bloodstream and impacts on blood sugar and weight, foods act the same for everyone.

There is, however, a variation of impact based on size. People of different sizes have different volumes of blood circulating through their bodies so the impact will vary based on the volume of blood in a person's body. A small female may have as little as five pints of blood circulating in her body, but a large male could have 10 pints or more circulating in his body.

If a small female, for example, ate the same size portions of a food I did, the impact on her blood glucose and weight would be proportionally greater than the impact on my blood sugar. If a 260-pound male—I'm 6 feet 2 inches and weigh about 180 pounds—ate the same food and portion sizes I did, the impact on his blood glucose and weight would be proportionally less than the impact on my blood glucose and weight. The speed with which the food converts to glucose and enters the bloodstream in all these cases would, however, be the same.

It's like putting a teaspoon of sugar in an 8 oz. glass of iced tea compared to putting a teaspoon of sugar in a 16 oz. glass of iced tea. The 8 oz. glass of iced tea would be twice as sweet. But the speed at which both glasses became sweeter is the same.

Aside from the variation I just explained, the results shown on my tests will be effectively the same for everyone. The slopes, the peaks, and the shaded area of the graphs will give a valid comparison of foods to each other. For example, if food "A" causes my blood sugar to rise *faster and more* than food "B", it will do the same for you. If food "C" causes my blood sugar to rise *more slowly and less* than food "D" it will do the same for you.

Not Just Memorizing What to Eat but Understanding Why

From 1985 through 1989, I chaired the US Olympic Committee's bids for the Olympic Winter Games. During those years, Anchorage was America's candidate.

I spoke around the world promoting Anchorage as a host city for the Winter Olympics. Our committee also hosted International Olympic Committee (IOC) members on visits to Anchorage.

One of the visitors we hosted was the IOC member from China. After his visit to Anchorage, he made a comment to me that I have never forgotten. As we were riding together to the airport for his return trip to China, he turned to me and said, "Mr. Chairman, I've heard you speak at many meetings around the world but I've forgotten much of what you said about Anchorage being an ideal host for the Olympic Winter Games. But when I saw your visual presentations, I remembered. Now that I've visited your city, I understand."

The visual presentations of the graphs will help you *remember*. But when you see your weight loss starting right away, *you'll understand*.

Understanding the Graphs

The graphs you are about to review have five major elements that you need to understand.

The horizontal axis of the graphs is measured across the bottom of the graph. It's labeled 0 through 90 minutes and represents the time in minutes that I measured the change in my blood glucose.

The vertical axis of the graphs is measured along the left side of the graph. It represents the rise in my blood glucose measured in milligrams per deciliter (mg/dl). Note that it starts at 100—a number in the midnormal range—not at zero.

The slope of the graphs is the angled line and represents speed of the rise in blood glucose.

- *The steeper the slope*, the faster the rise in blood glucose. Remember a fast rise in blood glucose usually means the glucose will be stored as a form of glucose or fat before you get a chance to burn it. That's bad for weight loss.

- *The flatter the slope*, the slower the rise in blood glucose. A slow rise usually means much of the glucose will be burned before it ever gets stored as fat and your body will have to burn existing fat to provide energy. That's good for weight loss.

The peak of the graphs shows how hard your pancreas is asked to work to get the glucose from that particular food out of the bloodstream and into the cells. This is very important for anyone who wants to avoid or reverse Type 2 diabetes

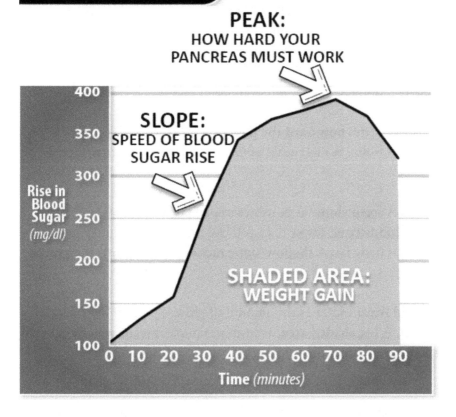

If you are overweight, you have probably already overworked your pancreas so you should do everything you can to lighten the workload of your pancreas. Please pay attention to the *peaks* of the graphs.

The shaded area of the graphs—The Crucial Measure of Weight gain or Weight loss.

The shaded area of the graphs shows the comparative weight gain the food or combination of foods will cause.

The faster the food causes your blood glucose to rise and the greater the rise, the *more weight* you will gain as illustrated by the large shaded area in some of the graphs. Avoid or minimize foods or drinks that create large shaded areas.

The slower the food causes your blood glucose to rise and the smaller the rise, as illustrated by a small shaded area in graphs, the *more likely your body will have to draw upon existing fat for energy and you will lose weight.*

Foods that create a smaller shaded area promote weight loss. If you eat those foods without changing your activity, *you will lose weight.* If you also increase your activity—which you will naturally do as you lose weight—you will lose weight even faster and find it easier to keep off.

Peak: Indicates **how hard the pancreas must work** to produce enough insulin. A high peak, as in this example, promotes Type 2 diabetes.

Slope: A **steep slope**, as in this example, **means glucose will enter your bloodstream faster** than you can burn it. Excess glucose will be stored as body fat. A **shallow slope means you can burn the glucose** before it is stored as body fat.

Shaded Area: Indicates the amount of glucose put into your bloodstream. **A big shaded area**, as in this example, **means weight gain**. A **small shaded area means weight loss**.

Why Counting Calories Hasn't Worked for America

While some weight-loss authors continue to promote counting calories, Americans keep getting fatter and fatter. Why? The reason is that not all calories are the same. As you review the graphs you'll see that 200 calories of protein, vegetables, and yes—even fat, will raise your blood glucose a lot less and contribute less to your weight gain than 200 calories of sweet or starchy carbs.

To illustrate, compare a 214-calorie Hershey bar (Graph 4) to three eggs cooked different ways (Graphs 42, 43, and 44), about 213 calories. Because a Hershey bar gets into your bloodstream much faster and ends with a much higher blood sugar, the contribution to weight—the gray area—is about six times greater than the gray area of three eggs. That means a single Hershey bar, or almost any candy bar, will cause much more weight gain than three eggs.

Another way to look at this comparison is that you can eat three eggs for breakfast for six days and gain about the same weight as one Hershey bar or other, similar candy bar.

Let's look at another comparison. Graph 5 show the impact of one of the most common bottles of Coke®. The 16.9 oz. size, which has, according to its label, 200 calories, is similar to most other sugared soft drinks of that size.

Compare Graph 5, a Coke to Graph 50, a 10 oz. piece of grilled Alaskan king salmon. That piece of salmon has 402 calories—twice as many calories as the Coke.

Now look at the impact on your weight (the shaded area of the two graphs). As you can see, despite the salmon having more than double the calories of the Coke®, the glucose creation and the weight gain created by the salmon is much smaller than those of the Coke®

Another fascinating way to look at this is to compare the 10 oz. piece of salmon to a Hershey bar that weighs less than 2 oz. Immediately following eating a 10 oz. piece of salmon, you will, of course, weigh 10 oz. more. The same for eating a 2 oz. candy bar. You will weigh 2 oz. more. But 24 to 36 hours later, when the waste of both have been excreted, the salmon will have created very little glucose and made a negligible impact on your weight, while the glucose from the Hershey bar will have been feeding your fat cells and have a greater impact on weight gain.

As you study the graphs, give special attention to the shaded area of each graph, you'll see over and over that it's not the calories but the food group and quality of food that counts.

One well-respected researcher and author, Gary Taubes, who wrote *Good Calories, Bad Calories*, explains convincingly that, "obesity is caused, not by the quantity of calories you eat but by the quality. Carbohydrates, particularly refined ones like white bread and pasta, raise insulin levels, promoting the storage of fat."

The results of my research show that *all starchy carbs* and sweet carbs raise insulin levels significantly and promote the growth of fat.

The only time you should pay attention to calories is when you are comparing foods in the same category. If you are comparing *starchy carbs to starchy carbs, sweet carbs to sweet carbs, fruit carbs to fruit carbs, veggie carbs to veggie carbs, protein to protein, and fat to fat,* looking at calories has some meaning.

The Value of Having Six Food Groups Instead of Just Three

As you review the graphs, it's most important that you go back and forth to compare graphs from food groups to graphs from other food groups and understand how the six different groups compare with one another.

No one can tell you how much *every* food you'll ever eat will contribute to your blood sugar and weight. Even if they could, no one could memorize all that and use it in a functional way.

Your primary goals should be to understand which food *groups* are the biggest contributors to high blood glucose and weight gain and which are not. You also need to have a general understanding of which foods are included in each group. By understanding those two factors, you can lose weight faster and maintain that lower weight more easily.

Applying the Graphs

By the time you finish reviewing these graphs you'll have a strong visual memory of which foods you must *minimize* to lower blood glucose and avoid weight gain, and which foods you can *maximize* to promote weight loss and lose body fat.

Once the graphs have found a secure place in your memory they will always be there. You'll always remember which food groups and which foods within those groups contribute more to blood sugar and weight gain, and which will contribute less to blood sugar and will result in weight loss.

Some Notes on the Graphs

As you review these graphs, you'll see that foods typical to breakfasts are measured and graphed more often than other meals.

There are two reasons I've done this. First, people tend to eat the same or similar foods most mornings for breakfast, so getting into a better pattern of eating is easier. Second, there seems to be more misinformation about healthy breakfast foods than about other meals. But because I've been testing for so long and so frequently, I know that whatever the timing of the meals, breakfast, lunch, dinner, or snacks, all the foods within the six food groups act similarly.

My Daily Feedback on the Impact of Foods on Weight

For most Americans, the only way they can get feedback on the impact of foods on weight is when they step on a scale. They can only speculate as to which of the foods they ate contributed to weight gain or loss. I get feedback on individual foods ten or more times a day and a summary result at the end of each day.

I know the information I'm sharing in these graphs can positively impact the lives of millions of people. I hope you are one.

Sweet Carbohydrates

I'm going to start with sweet carbs. We all know they make your blood glucose go up and contribute substantially to weight gain. No surprise there. But these graphs will give readers perspective on how much and how fast this happens. It also gives a point of reference for the rest of the food categories.

Here's a review of foods in this category:

Sweetened soft drinks, candy bars, cakes, pies, donuts, sweet rolls, sweet toppings for ice creams, chocolates, caramels, other sweetened candies, sweet desserts. We all know by now that too much sugar is a villain. Then what about all the *sugar-free* candies? Are they okay? They taste just like regular candy. But look closely at the label. You'll see that many of those items are sweetened with high-fructose corn syrup or with other sweeteners like sucrose—not much different from cane sugars, but a little more concentrated…and therefore worse for you.

Don't think you're doing yourself a favor by eating *sugar-free* candy. It only means the manufacturers have likely used concentrated sweeteners other than sugar. Both regular candy and sugar-free candy are items that you need to start minimizing or better yet, eliminating. This is, of course, not new information but if you do all the other things I'll propose and still eat lots of sweets, you're not going to make the progress you need or want.

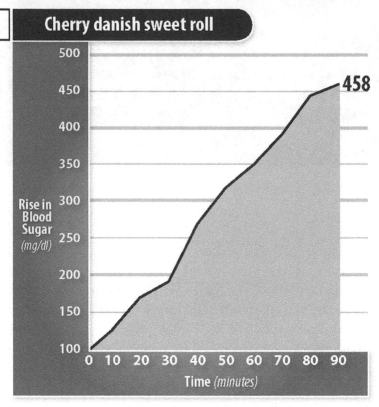

1 **Cherry danish sweet roll**

Rise in Blood Sugar *(mg/dl)*

458

Time *(minutes)*

Total Calories – 440

Cherry Danish

This is my record holder for increasing my blood sugar. It went from 100 to 458 mg/dl in 90 minutes. This caused a net blood sugar rise* of 358 mg/dl in 90 minutes. As you'll see when you review other graphs, this is a huge rise and a great contributor to weight.

Because this Cherry Danish causes a big increase in glucose 358mg/DL from 110 to 458 (the peak), and because it goes in very fast (the slope), it will cause a great increase in weight (represented by the shaded area). Evaluate each of the graphs in this way: Look at the peak, the

---

* *Notice that the net blood glucose rise is 100 points less than my final blood glucose on the graph. The reason is, of course, that all my blood sugars are indexed to start at 100, which is within the generally accepted normal levels, so the starting point must be subtracted from the finishing blood sugar to get the net rise.*

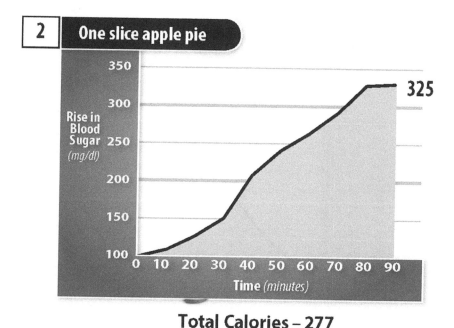

2 | **One slice apple pie**

Rise in Blood Sugar *(mg/dl)*

325

Time *(minutes)*

Total Calories – 277

slope and the shaded area. You're looking for foods that have the smallest and slowest increases in blood glucose (the flattest slope) and the smallest shaded area (the weight increase area).

Apple Pie

This is another big rise in blood glucose. This blood glucose rise is typical of most pies. Whether you cut out desserts like this, eat them much less frequently, or dramatically reduce portion size will be up to you. The important thing right now is to lock this visual in your mind. Most pies and cakes will act similarly to this. Though I eat a small piece or small slice of cake only about three or four times a year, their combination of sweet carbs and starchy carbs have always caused the biggest rises in my blood glucose and weight. The few times I do eat a pie, I must give myself a huge infusion of insulin that is often larger than the infusion for the complete meal preceding it. That means the pie or cake would raise my blood glucose more and make me fatter than all the rest of the food on my plate combined.

Having a dessert on special occasions is a part of life. Just don't make it a habit.

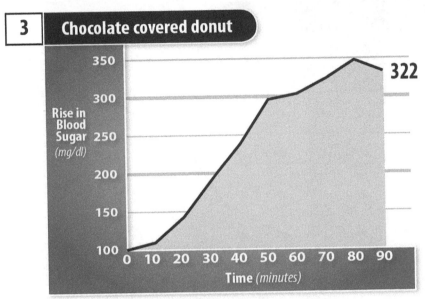

3 | **Chocolate covered donut**

322

Rise in Blood Sugar (mg/dl)

Time (minutes)

Total Calories – 276

Chocolate-Covered Donut

Here's another food that has an impact even greater than most would expect. Donuts are a common breakfast habit for many people. If you eat a donut or a sweet roll for breakfast and wonder why you're gaining weight, compare this graph to other breakfast choices shown in later graphs.

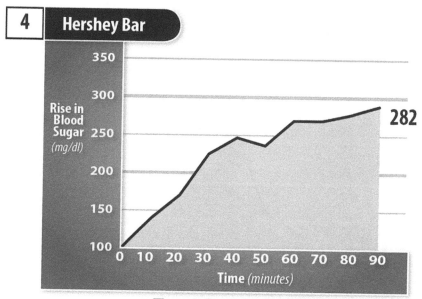

4 | **Hershey Bar**

Rise in Blood Sugar (mg/dl)

282

Total Calories – 214

Hershey Bar®

I've included a Hershey bar graph because it is such a common candy bar and people can relate to it. Both the slope and the impact are less than the first three graphs but still significant. A Hershey bar has 214 calories. Compare this graph to eggs (Graphs 42, 43, and 44). Three large eggs have 210 to 214 calories total but have a much smaller impact on blood glucose and weight gain than a Hershey bar does. This illustrates why calories are only pertinent if foods from the same group are compared.

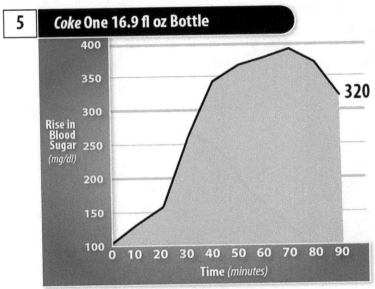

5 | *Coke* One 16.9 fl oz Bottle

Rise in Blood Sugar *(mg/dl)*

320

Time *(minutes)*

Total Calories – 200

Coke

I've included a graph of a 500ml (16.9 fl.oz.) bottle of Coca Cola, which is the most common size I've found in stores. It gets into your bloodstream very quickly, which is bad because you will not likely burn that glucose before it is stored in your liver as glycogen and around your body as body fat. If you regularly drink any sugared soft drinks or similar drinks, such as Slurpee's, you will not lose weight. You must stop that unhealthy, fat-building habit. Do not drink artificially sweetened "diet" soft drinks. First, they will continue to feed your sweet need, which will go away in about three months if you stop now. Second, neither you nor I understand the impact all the chemicals have on our health. And third, all the folks I know who drink diet soft drinks are overweight. The zero-calorie diet soft drinks may not cause overweight, but observation certainly shows they are not solving it.

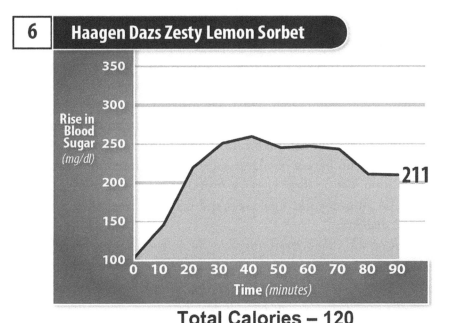

6 | **Haagen Dazs Zesty Lemon Sorbet**

Total Calories – 120

Ice Cream or Sorbet

I'm sorry to report that ice cream in its various forms is a big contributor to blood sugar elevation and weight gain. The combination of sweet carbs and fat is not good. You'll learn later in this book why you should avoid eating ice cream late in the evening. If you really love ice cream—doesn't everyone—and can't do without it, eat it earlier in the day and do everything you can to minimize it. For a smaller impact, it's best to get out of the habit of any ice cream. Once in a while, I eat Haagen Daz Zesty Lemon Sorbet. It does have a lot of sugar but does not combine it with fat—which combination is bad for anyone who doesn't want to gain weight.

For this test, I ate about one half of a half-pint container (1/4 pint) which is a lot for me. When I do eat it, I typically eat just a tablespoon at a time so a pint may last me three weeks to a month. But it is very refreshing and tasty.

Conclusions Regarding the Sweet Carbohydrates Group

We all know sweets are a big contributor to high blood sugars and significant weight gain. But after you review all the graphs, return and look at these sweet carb graphs, you'll see just how significant the blood glucose increases and weight gains are compared to other food groups.

You can eat three eggs for breakfast for four days and gain less weight than you'll gain having one large sugared soft drink or one sweet roll. In addition, eating three eggs for breakfast for a week puts a lot less strain on an overworked pancreas and will help you avoid or reverse Type 2 diabetes.

Note: Remember, the determining factor for weight loss is how much glucose is created in your bloodstream and how fast that glucose gets into your bloodstream. Calories are not a determining factor for weight loss unless you compare calories in the same food groups.

In this example, the Coke has 200 calories and three eggs five times a week would total about 1,200 calories. That calorie count is totally irrelevant. The total contribution to weight is how much glucose gets into your bloodstream and how fast it goes in. The eggs are slow going in as glucose and create only a small amount of glucose compared to the Coke, which gets into your bloodstream very fast and creates a lot of glucose. The resulting gray area of the eggs, representing weight gain, is small—less than one-fifth of the gray area of the Coke or any sugared soft drink of that size.

Now let's look at the next food group, starchy carbs.

Starchy Carbohydrates

My next category of foods based on the speed of absorption and total impact on blood glucose and weight gain is starchy carbohydrates. This is a food group that you need to minimize significantly if you want to lose weight. As a reminder, here are some examples of foods I include in this category:

waffles

pancakes

breakfast cereals

white breads

rolls

bagels

buns

multigrain breads

whole-grain bread is somewhat better than multigrain or white breads but should still be minimized

muffins

spaghetti

lasagna

pasta

tortillas

rice

brown rice is slightly better than white rice

Other starchy carbs to minimize are snacks like:

potato chips   Cheetos   tortilla chips

The two snacks in this category I recommend are Crunchmaster© Rice Crackers and Organic Triscuits. Add butter to both. This will allow you to burn the small amount of blood glucose they create before that glucose can be stored as fat.

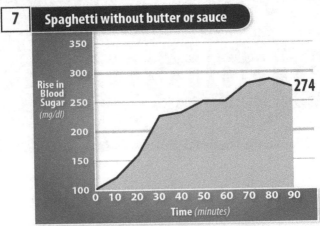

Total Calories – 220

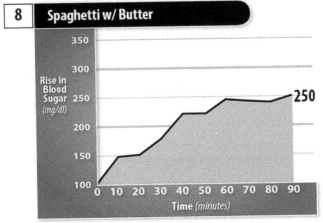

Total Calories – 310

Spaghetti

These graphs show the impact of a starchy carbohydrate (spaghetti) with and without butter. The purpose in this graph is to illustrate the blood glucose and weight gain impact of a starchy carb alone and the same starchy carb with fat (butter). Note how blood glucose goes up more slowly when butter is added to the spaghetti. If I had tested for more than 90 minutes you would see that the spaghetti with butter would continue to raise blood sugar longer than spaghetti without butter. Either with or without butter, this is a big contributor to weight gain.

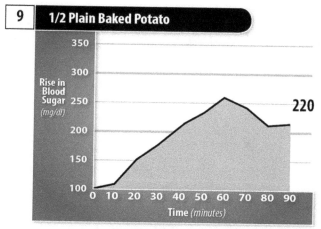

9 1/2 Plain Baked Potato

Rise in Blood Sugar (mg/dl)

220

Time (minutes)

Total Calories – 100

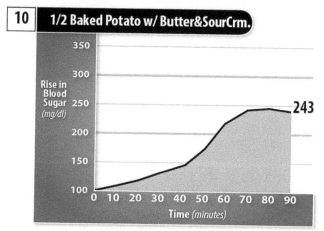

10 1/2 Baked Potato w/ Butter&SourCrm.

Rise in Blood Sugar (mg/dl)

243

Time (minutes)

Total Calories – 235

Potatoes

Note how the potatoes with butter and sour cream enter the bloodstream more slowly. This gives you a better chance to burn the glucose before it gets stored as body fat. We would all be better off if we ate half as much potato with twice as much butter and sour cream. You'll see what I mean when I get to the "fat" graphs. I'll also address cholesterol and the changing way medical professionals are evaluating HDL and LDL cholesterol.

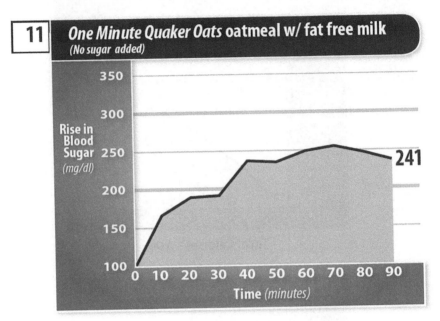

11 **One Minute Quaker Oats oatmeal w/ fat free milk** *(No sugar added)*

Total Calories – 230

Oatmeal

Oatmeal is widely considered a healthy breakfast and although that may be true, it is not a good weight-loss breakfast. It is slightly better for weight loss than the other cereals that I show in the coming graphs. However, as you continue with this chapter, you will see other choices that are better for blood glucose control and weight loss.

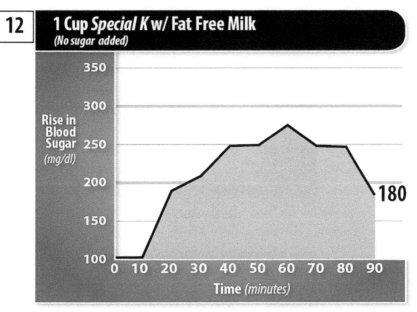

12 **1 Cup *Special K* w/ Fat Free Milk**
(No sugar added)

Total Calories – 200

Cereal

Most cereals seem to identify about the same range of calories in their nutrition facts—usually between 100 and 130, but as you will continue to see, calories and blood glucose, and calories and weight gain are not always related. Some foods with more calories have smaller impacts on blood glucose and weight gain than other foods with fewer calories. When you compare these cereal graphs with graphs of three eggs which have more calories, you'll begin to understand that statement.

I don't eat much cereal because of the big impact on my blood sugar and weight but I chose Total and Special K to test because they looked the healthiest from the box information. The results of these tests are quite consistent with my general experience with many different cereals. Of the cereals that I have tested, General Mills' Fiber One has the least impact on my blood sugar and therefore on weight gain, but even with that cereal you need to keep the portion size small.

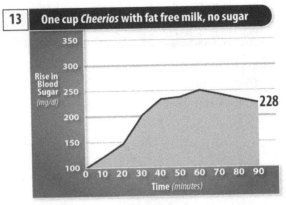

13 One cup *Cheerios* with fat free milk, no sugar

Net blood sugar rise – 128

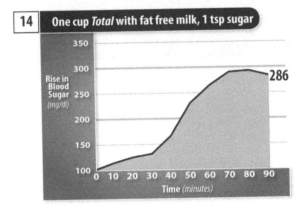

14 One cup *Total* with fat free milk, 1 tsp sugar

Net blood sugar rise – 186

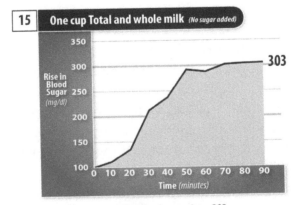

15 One cup Total and whole milk *(No sugar added)*

Net blood sugar rise – 203

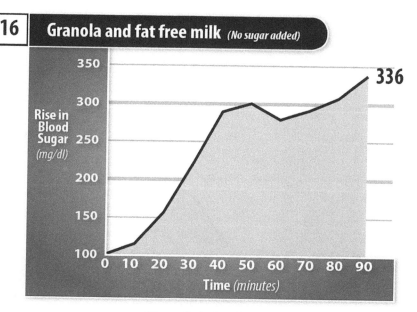

16 **Granola and fat free milk** *(No sugar added)*

350

300

Rise in Blood Sugar 250
(mg/dl)

200

150

100

336

0 10 20 30 40 50 60 70 80 90

Time *(minutes)*

Total Calories – 406

Granola

I don't recall ever eating granola as a breakfast cereal before this test, so I didn't know what to expect. But, like many Americans, I always associated granola with good health, so I was at first surprised by the results showing big and fast increases in blood glucose.

After reflecting on the test, I concluded that's exactly why granola is popular among runners. A small bowl of granola is ideal for giving your body a large influx of glucose and fiber without much volume of food. Perfect if you're going on a five-mile training run after eating it but not good if you're going to the office or sitting at a desk after eating it.

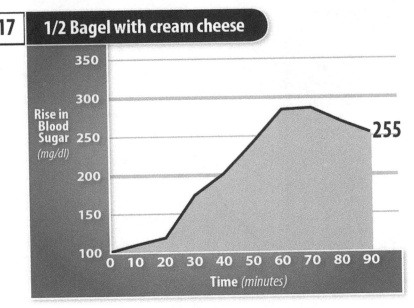

17 | **1/2 Bagel with cream cheese**

Rise in Blood Sugar (mg/dl)

350
300
250 — 255
200
150
100

Time (minutes)
0 10 20 30 40 50 60 70 80 90

Total Calories – 219

Bagels

Bagels seem to be a food that people who are health conscious eat. I've often heard folks say with a certain modicum of self-pride, "I usually just have a bagel and cream cheese for breakfast." With that statement in mind, I tested, not a full bagel, but one-half bagel with cream cheese and then a bagel without cream cheese or butter. If this is what a half bagel does, think about the impact of a full bagel. You'd be getting into Cherry Danish territory.

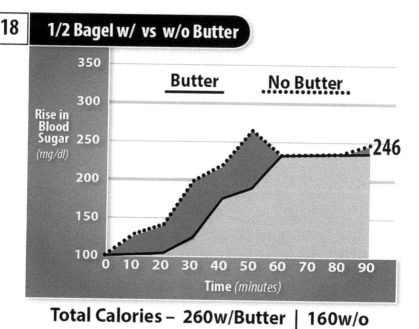

On Graph 18, the light gray area is a bagel with butter. The dark gray added to the light gray is a bagel without butter. The butter slows down the entry of glucose into the bloodstream and gives you slightly more opportunity to burn the glucose before it gets stored. The only time you should eat a bagel for breakfast is if you are going to exercise right after breakfast or walk to work, then only a half bagel. Better choices for breakfast are coming up.

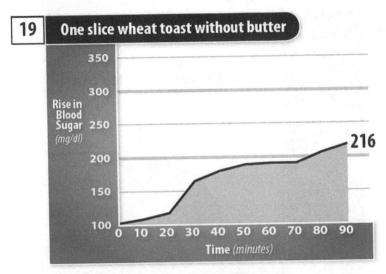

19 One slice wheat toast without butter

216

Total Calories – 69

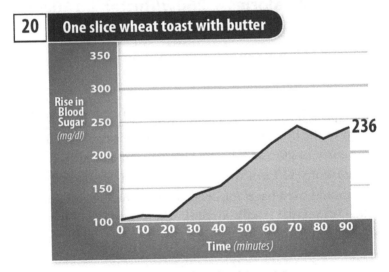

20 One slice wheat toast with butter

236

Total Calories – 90

I've also gradually reduced the number of bread products that I eat because of their discouragingly high increases in my blood glucose and therefore weight.

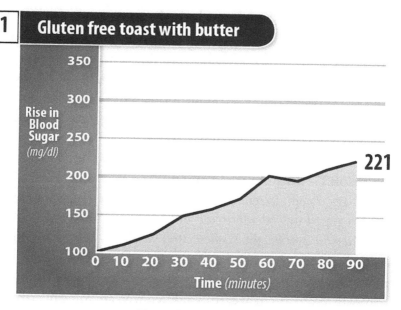

21 **Gluten free toast with butter**

Total Calories – 91

Gluten-Free Toast

Gluten-free toast is not something I'm familiar with nor have I eaten it prior to the tests graphed below, so I can't say that the few tests I took are absolute certainties, but the corn starch and tapioca starch in gluten-free bread appear to have a slightly smaller impact on my blood sugar than the wheat in other breads.

Conclusions on Starchy Carbohydrates

It's been my experience as a result of thousands of blood sugar tests that starchy carbs will raise my blood sugar almost as much as sweet carbs. I'm not suggesting that sweet carbs and starchy carbs are equivalent in terms of general health. I'm confident that starchy carbs are better, but if you want to lower blood glucose, and lose weight, then dramatically reducing starchy carbs is absolutely necessary.

A Note on Healthy, Active Children

This is a good point to remind readers that the eating suggestions I make here are geared toward adults and not young, active, growing children. If children are overweight or obese, they would do well by following the advice in my eating recommendations, but if they're of normal weight, active, and growing, these recommendations are not for them— especially with regard to starchy carbs. Children who are going out to play for three or four hours after breakfast will do fine with cereal and toast but if they're going to sit in a classroom or in front of a computer or television they should cut back on starchy carbs for breakfast.

Once you see the graphs of how the next four categories of foods act you'll begin to be able to visually compare how much starchy carbs and sweet carbs contribute to high blood glucose and weight gain in contrast to the food groups that follow.

Fruit Carbohydrates

The foods in this category are quite obvious. Everyone knows what fruits are:

apples

oranges

mangos

pineapples

bananas

cantaloupe

watermelons

peaches

pears

berries

etc.

Fruit carbs are generally better than sweet carbs and starchy carbs in terms of blood glucose and weight control. They also are known to provide more healthful nutrients than the first two categories. But are they a free ride? Can you eat as much fruit as you wish without significant blood sugar increases and weight gain? No! You can't. You need to practice moderation with fruits.

I'll start with the fruits that have the highest impact on blood sugar and weight gain and move to fruits with lower impact on blood sugar and weight.

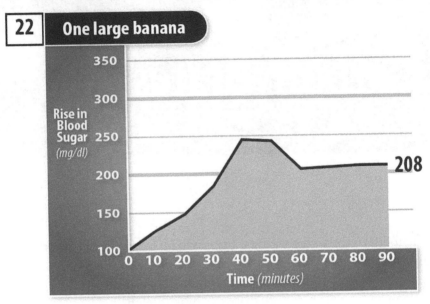

22 | **One large banana**

Rise in Blood Sugar (mg/dl)

208

Time (minutes)

Total Calories – 121

Bananas

Bananas have the highest impact on my blood sugar of the common fruits that I eat. Pineapples raised my blood sugar more than bananas do so I haven't eaten them for years. That, I think, is obvious to most people because of the extraordinary sweetness of pineapples. But bananas don't have that sweet taste so their impact would be hard for someone to tell just based on taste. In the graph, you'll see the impact of a banana on blood glucose and its contribution to weight gain are big. Consider for a moment what would happen if you added a banana to the cereal graphs that you just saw. That combination will create a huge impact on blood glucose and weight gain.

Regular (not sweetened) cereal with a banana is okay for your kids who are still growing and maybe going out to play after eating breakfast. But not for adults who want to lose weight.

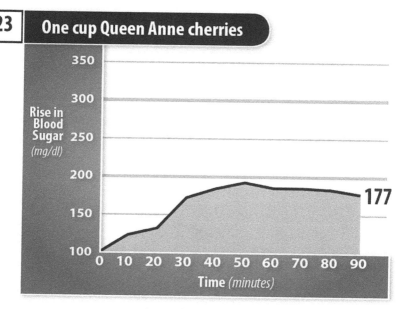

23 | **One cup Queen Anne cherries**

Rise in Blood Sugar (mg/dl)

177

Time (minutes)

Total Calories – 91

Queen Anne Cherries

I eat a small to moderate number of cherries—usually Queen Anne or Bing cherries. Cherries have only a moderate impact on blood sugar. Notice how the gray area, which represents weight gain is getting smaller. This graph shows the weight gain of one cup. If you eat ½ cup your blood glucose rise would be about 38 mg/Dl instead of 77 mg/Dl. They're a great snack if you eat ½ cup or less at a sitting.

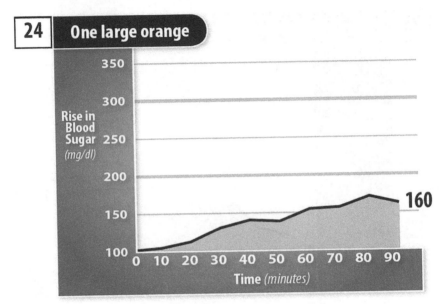

Total Calories – 87

Oranges

Oranges are in the middle of fruits in terms of blood sugar impact and weight contribution. However, do not make the mistake of thinking orange juice is good for weight loss. As you will see in coming graphs, it is not. Oranges themselves are okay but not as good as the fruits to come.

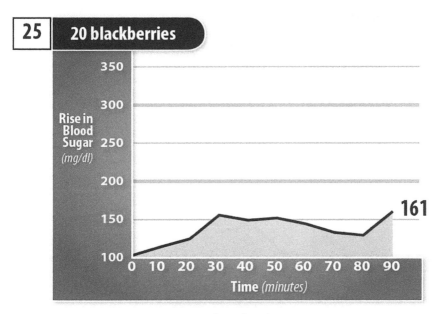

25 **20 blackberries**

Total Calories – 62

Blackberries

Blackberries have about the same impact as oranges. They are not too bad in terms of blood glucose, but you still won't want to splurge on them. Ten to 20 blackberries are a good snack with little impact on your weight.

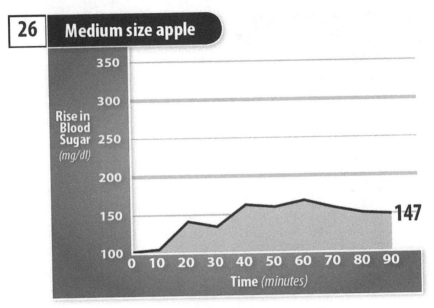

Total Calories – 95

Apples

Apples are good; not too much impact on blood sugar or weight and not much likelihood of overindulging by eating two or three apples. This test is a whole apple. A half apple is proportionally better for weight loss than a whole apple.

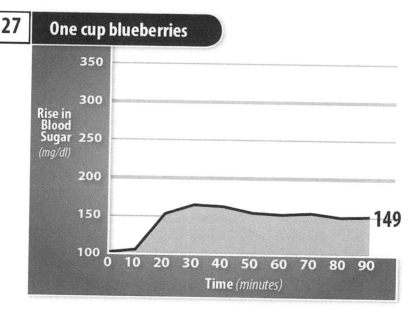

27 | **One cup blueberries**

Total Calories – 85

Blueberries

This graph shows one cup, but that's a lot of blueberries. You'll find that ½ cup is plenty and will raise your blood glucose by only about 25mg/Dl instead of 49. Not only will blueberries have little influence on your blood glucose and weight but everything I've read praises them for all their healthy ingredients.

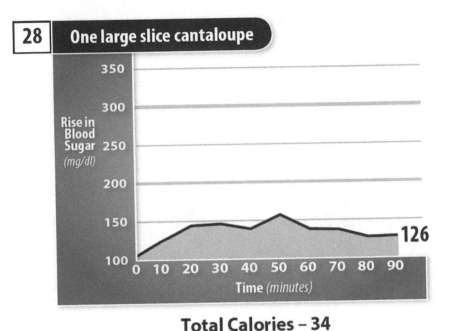

28 One large slice cantaloupe

Rise in Blood Sugar (mg/dl)

350
300
250
200
150
100

126

0 10 20 30 40 50 60 70 80 90

Time (minutes)

Total Calories – 34

Cantaloupe

Cantaloupe in season is a wonderful breakfast fruit for weight loss and a good, healthy weight-loss dessert for lunch and dinner. This is a fruit that because of its sweet taste, I expected to have a greater impact on my blood glucose than it does. Once I realized what a small impact it had on my blood glucose and weight, I began eating it regularly—when it is in season—at any meal. It's a great weight-loss fruit.

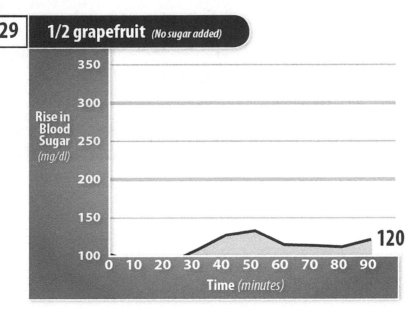

29 **1/2 grapefruit** *(No sugar added)*

Total Calories – 52

Grapefruit

This graph disagrees with some things I've read about grapefruit causing high rises in blood sugar but my 40 years of experience with grapefruit is consistent with what this graph shows. By the way, I haven't put sugar on anything or in anything since I got diabetes and I don't miss it. I don't use artificial sweeteners at all because I believe that contributes to maintaining a taste and desire for sweeter things.

Conclusions on the Fruit Carbohydrate Group

Despite the vitamins, minerals, and general health benefits fruits offer, they are not a free ride. In other words, in general, they contribute moderately to increased blood sugar and slight weight gain. Anyone trying to lose weight needs to be moderate in the consumption of fruits— especially pineapples and bananas.

Fruit Juices

Still within my category of fruit carbohydrates are fruit juices. Following are graphs for three of the most common fruit juices: apple juice, orange juice, and grapefruit juice. I've also tested and graphed my "go-to" juice, V-8, which will give an interesting point of reference.

In the fruit juice graphs, it's important to note how fast the juices increase blood glucose. Because of these fast increases, pay special attention to the volume of the gray shaded area reflecting weight gain created by the fruit juices as compared to V-8 juice, which has a significantly smaller gray shaded area because of its slower and lower blood glucose increase. V-8 juice, therefore, is a healthy promoter of weight loss.

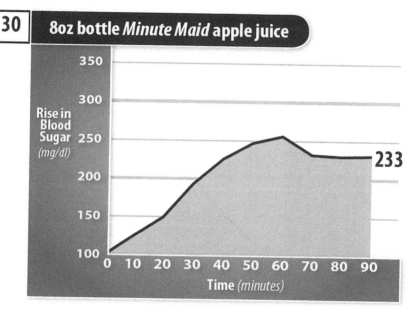

30 | **8oz bottle *Minute Maid* apple juice**

Rise in Blood Sugar *(mg/dl)*

233

Time *(minutes)*

Total Calories – 110

Apple Juice

Note that the net blood sugar increase from apple juice is 133 mg/dl. That approaches three times the 47 mg/dl blood sugar increase of a medium-size apple (Graph 26). But even more important than that, note the huge difference in the volume of the shaded area of the apple juice compared to an apple. This is a dramatic visualization of the bigger contribution to weight gain of the juice compared to the fruit itself.

Also compare this 8 oz. bottle of apple juice to the Coke graph which is 16 oz. The Coke peaks out at nearly 400 mg/dl. If this were a 16 oz. bottle of apple juice, it would have peaked at about 500 mg./dl. Comparing an equal amount of apple juice and Coke, the apple juice will raise your blood glucose more than Coke and equally fast, therefore adding more body fat.

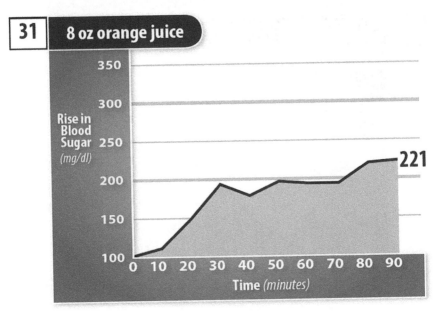

31 8 oz orange juice

Total Calories – 102

Orange Juice

Orange juice provides a similar comparison, though not as dramatic as apple juice. The net rise in blood sugar caused by orange juice is 121 mg/dl compared to 60 for a large orange. Once again though, because the orange juice increases blood glucose fast, the shaded area representing the juice's contribution to weight gain is significantly larger than the orange itself.

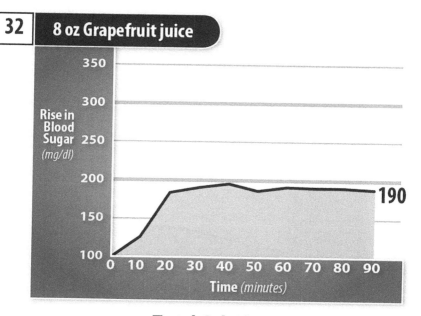

32 | **8 oz Grapefruit juice**

190

Total Calories – 88

Grapefruit Juice

Now compare grapefruit juice to ½ grapefruit (Graph 29). Not only does the juice cause a much bigger rise than the grapefruit itself, but because it causes such a fast rise, it goes into your bloodstream faster than you can use it and much of the excess glucose it causes—just like apple juice and orange juice—will end up being stored in the liver or as body fat. This comparison also shows the net blood sugar rise for ½ grapefruit of 20 mg/dl compared to a net rise of the juice of 90. Now some will argue that I should have compared a full grapefruit to 8 ounces of juice. They may be right but my goal here is to compare typical portions. I don't ever recall seeing anyone eating two grapefruit halves in a restaurant, but I often see folks drinking 8 ounces or more of whatever juice they ordered. Even if I were to double the grapefruit portion, it would still be less than half of the increase in blood glucose of the juice.

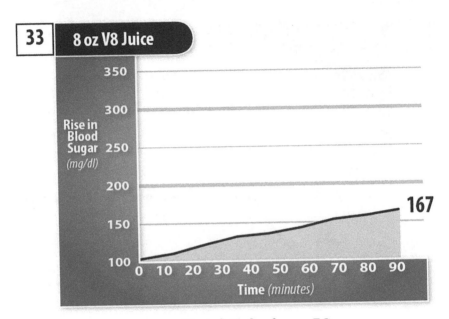

33 8 oz V8 Juice

Rise in
Blood
Sugar *(mg/dl)*

167

Time *(minutes)*

Total Calories – 50

V-8 Juice

This is not a fruit juice. It's a vegetable juice but I've included it in this category to compare it to other juices.

This graph is a good illustration of the value of foods or liquids that cause slower rises in blood sugar. In this case the V-8 juice reaches a lower level than the other juices do and it reaches that level much more slowly as shown in these graphs. The slow rise in glucose means less of the glucose created by V-8 juice will be stored since you'll be burning it as it enters. You won't be able to burn the glucose from the other juices as fast as they go in so the excess glucose will be stored as glycogen in your liver and then as body fat.

I can rarely get V-8 in restaurants but it's the juice of choice for me at home. For the past few years, I've been diluting about a third to a half of a large glass of V-8 juice with two thirds of a glass of Pellegrino, Perrier, or Signature Sparkling Mineral Water. It's now not only my favorite breakfast drink but also a very refreshing midday or evening drink.

I also mix V-8 with whole milk in a coffee cup. Put it in the microwave for 2 minutes and it becomes a tasty and healthy tomato-like soup with lunch. It also substitutes for a second cup of coffee in the morning.

V-8 juice is a good friend of weight loss and a healthy go-to juice for anyone who wants to lose weight.

V-8 juice also has a low-sodium version for those who have high blood pressure. You will find, however, that by following Glucose Control Eating©, your blood pressure will go down dramatically as you lose weight.

Conclusions Regarding Fruit Juices

Diluting your morning fruit juice is one of the easiest actions you can take. Your weight loss will, of course, depend on how much juice you drink now. The more juice you drink now, the more weight you will lose when you start diluting your juices.

Whether you dilute your juice with sparkling water, tap water, or bottled water, you'll soon find the diluted juice becoming an easy and refreshing pattern that will become a habit in no time. It's one of those small actions that will make a big difference over time.

Vegetable Carbohydrates

Now we're getting into the good stuff. Your mother was right—eat your vegetables. She probably told you they would make you healthy but what she didn't know is how little they contribute to blood glucose and how much they can contribute to weight loss. To the extent that you can eat more of the foods that have little impact on your blood glucose and less of the foods that have greater impact on your blood glucose, you will lose weight even if you're eating the same volume of food as you did previously. If you eat more vegetables and a smaller volume of starchy *and* sweet carbs, your pounds will just melt off.

As you will see, vegetables are the carbohydrate group that has the smallest impact on your blood glucose.

You will see in the graphs how vegetables create small amounts of glucose and promote weight loss. You'll also see in the graphs that you can put all the butter you want on vegetables with almost no impact on blood glucose. Butter makes the already small amount of glucose created by the vegetable go into the bloodstream more slowly and allows you more time to burn the glucose before it turns to body fat. Putting butter on vegetables will also keep you from getting hungry as quickly (more on that later). The added bonus is the butter makes vegetables taste better, so you'll eat more vegetables. That's your goal, eat more of the good stuff, less of the bad stuff.

Take a minute now and go back to the sweet and starchy carbs graphs and compare them to the following veggies carb graphs. Compare how fast sweet and starchy carbs get into your bloodstream, how high they go and finally compare the gray area. The faster a food goes in and the more glucose it creates, the greater the shaded area and the more weight it adds.

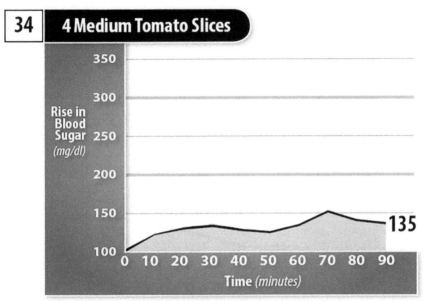

34 | **4 Medium Tomato Slices**

Total Calories – 20

Tomatoes

Contrary to some advice, tomatoes are good for keeping blood glucose and weight down. Be careful of tomato soup, ketchup, and some salsas, which often have sugar added.

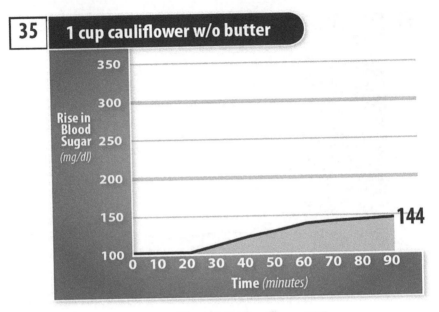

35 | 1 cup cauliflower w/o butter

Total Calories – 27

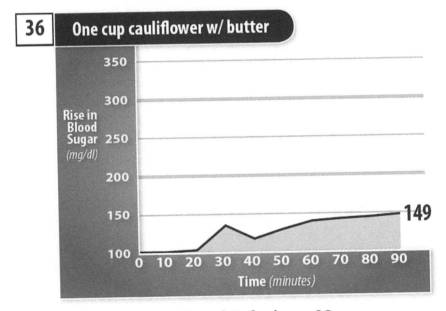

36 | One cup cauliflower w/ butter

Total Calories – 48

Cauliflower

Here's an illustration of the very minor impact of fat (in this case butter) when combined with veggie carbs. You can see by comparing the two graphs that eating cauliflower with butter creates an almost imperceptible impact on blood glucose.

It took me years to figure out that *butter on vegetables* has almost no impact on blood glucose. The low, slow rise in blood glucose caused by vegetables combined with the even lower, slower rise caused by butter makes the combination of the two a friend of weight loss and good health.

Once you finish this book and understand that butter is a good—but conditional—friend of weight loss, you will find yourself eating a lot more vegetables because they simply taste better with butter or butter-based sauces.

Because you've been told all your life, "If you don't want to get fat, don't eat fat" it may be hard for you to buy into butter as a friend of weight loss. I will spend a lot of time in the next two chapters discussing the evolving science of the role of fat and butter on good health—including improving the ratio of good to bad cholesterol.

It took me almost 25 years of testing before I figured out that butter *is* a conditional friend of weight loss. When butter is combined with vegetables (except corn and potatoes) and protein like halibut, salmon, crab, lobster, shrimp, trout, rockfish, clams, and mussels, it contributes almost nothing to weight gain, no matter how much you eat. Eat all you want of those foods and put as much butter as you like on them.

Here's the *conditional* part of butter as a conditional contributor to weight loss. *Butter on starchy carbs* like bread, toast, muffins, or biscuits, rice, pasta, and spaghetti is a big contributor to weight gain. If you have a meal with butter on vegetables or protein but also in that meal you have starchy carbs, you will negate the weight-loss benefit of the butter on vegetables. Further, if you have a meal of vegetables and protein with butter and follow it with a sweet dessert, you increase dramatically the weight gain of the dessert alone.

Avoid butter if you are going to include starchy carbs in a meal or if you are going to follow a meal with a sweet dessert.

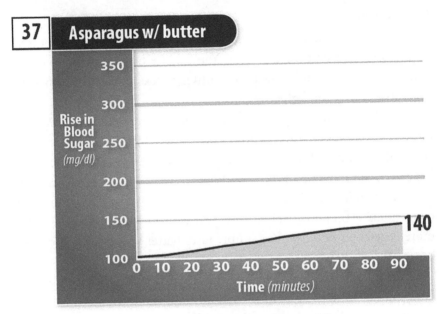

37 **Asparagus w/ butter**

Total Calories – 48

Asparagus

Asparagus with butter has about the same minimal impact on blood glucose and weight as cauliflower with butter.

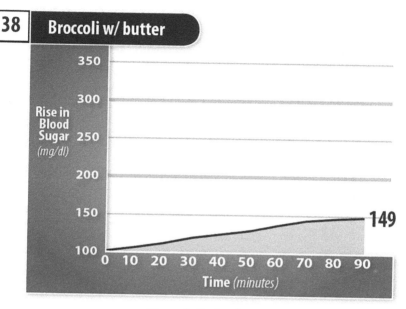

38 | **Broccoli w/ butter**

Total Calories – 51

Broccoli

This graph shows broccoli's insignificant impact on blood sugar and weight gain. When I discovered the small impact of putting butter on vegetables, I began eating more vegetables. You will probably eat more vegetables too. It's a good example of eating more of the good weight-loss foods and less of the weight-gain foods.

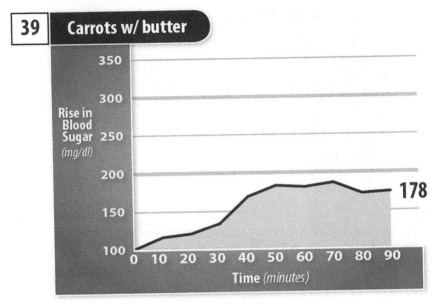

39 | **Carrots w/ butter**

Total Calories – 71

Carrots

You can see by the graph that the impact of carrots on blood sugar and weight is higher than that of the previous vegetables, but not as high as corn and potatoes, and certainly not as high as starchy or sweet carbs.

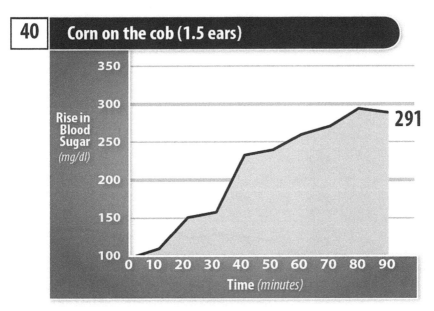

40 | Corn on the cob (1.5 ears)

Rise in Blood Sugar (mg/dl)

291

Time (minutes)

Total Calories – 232.5

Corn

When I said, "With just a few exceptions, eat more vegetables and you'll lose weight," corn is one of those exceptions. Although corn is a vegetable carbohydrate, it acts more like a starchy carbohydrate. Take a look at this graph and compare it to the other veggie carbs. Like starchy carbs, corn creates a high amount of blood glucose and therefore insulin demand which means more weight gain.

Moderate corn in your eating lifestyle.

Like corn, potatoes also act more like a starchy carb than a veggie carb. They are a good source of vitamin C and potassium but are also contributors to increased blood glucose and therefore weight. Don't eliminate them from Glucose Control Eating© but rather cut back and moderate the butter on corn or the gravy you put on potatoes.

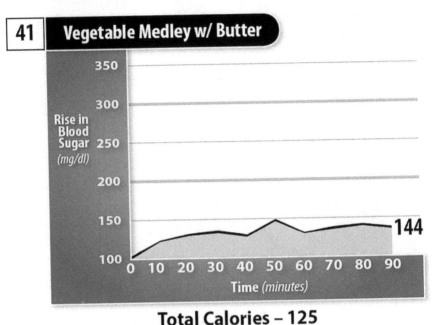

41 **Vegetable Medley w/ Butter**

Rise in Blood Sugar (mg/dl)

144

Time (minutes)

Total Calories – 125

This vegetable medley consists of broccoli, cauliflower, and carrots

Conclusions on Vegetable Carbohydrate Group

The message from these graphs is that vegetables in general have very little impact on blood glucose and promote weight loss.

Adding butter to vegetables has only a tiny impact on blood sugar.

Because neither vegetables nor fat trigger a rise in blood glucose. The combination of vegetables and fat is a good mixture in a healthy weight-loss meal.

I've had many people tell me that reducing the quantity of food they eat is very difficult and they always feel hungry. The best way to solve that problem and lose weight without feeling hungry is to eat more vegetables and be free with butter...and don't forget to drink plenty of V-8 juice mixed with mineral water.

In the next graphic section, I cover two other food groups that will be instrumental in your weight loss: protein and fat.

Protein and Fat

I've combined protein and fat because very few common foods are exclusively fat. The two most common foods that derive all their calories from fat are butter (100 calories per serving—all from fat) and olive oil (125 calories per serving—all from fat). Wow, with those calories from fat, they must add a lot of body fat. Right? No. Wrong in most cases!

Remember that I said fat is a "friend of weight loss, but a conditional friend." You're about to find out why I call fat a "conditional" friend. In the next sections of the graphs, you're going to see in more detail than previously which food groups and foods you can combine with fat to promote weight loss, and which combinations of food groups and foods when combined with fat will promote weight gain.

Once again compare the small, slow increases in the upcoming graphs to the big increases in blood glucose and weight caused by sweet carbs, starchy carbs, and fruit juices.

First some breakfast foods containing both protein and fat

Three Large Eggs

Large eggs have about 70-85 calories each—depending on the size of the eggs— so three eggs have about 210-255 calories. That's more than the number of calories in a Hershey bar—210 calories. Now compare the Hershey bar graph (Graph 4) to these three egg graphs (Graphs 42, 43, and 44). These three graphs show how slowly the eggs convert to glucose and how small that conversion to glucose is. It very strongly illustrates the point that calories are not a good indicator of impact on weight gain. Take special note of how small the gray shaded area in the graphs are which you now know represents potential weight gain.

Comparing the shaded area on the Hershey bar® graph with the shaded area of the egg graphs, you can see that one Hershey bar® will result in a weight gain many times greater than three eggs. To put it in functional terms, you can eat a breakfast of three eggs, four or five days in a row before you will have the same impact on weight as eating one Hershey bar® or other similar candy bar.

Make the same comparison between eggs and cereal (Graphs 12, 13, 14, and 15). When you compare the size of the shaded areas, you can visually see that you will gain around four times as much weight from cereal as you will from three eggs.

When you embrace Glucose Control Eating©, you will also learn that you will not get hungry again nearly as quickly as you will with cereal.

Remember when you hear, you forget; when you see, you remember; but when you experience your weight loss, you will understand.

It's a good illustration of the value of foods that enter your bloodstream more slowly. Remember, the slower the food's entry into your bloodstream, the more likely you'll burn it before you store it. Even with a minimal amount of activity, that small potential weight gain will become a weight loss. You'll also note very little difference between poached eggs and boiled or fried eggs. The boiled and fried eggs include butter and the poached eggs don't—thus the difference in calories.

As an aside, I eat three boiled eggs every morning and add about a tablespoon of butter to the eggs as I mash them with a fork. If you choose two eggs instead of three, the impact on your blood glucose and weight will be about 1/3 less.

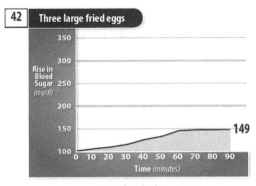

Total Calories – 276

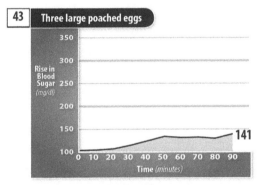

Total Calories – 213

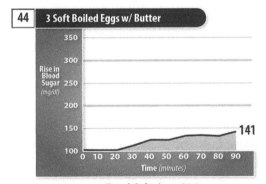

Total Calories – 234

Adding butter to eggs and adding vegetables with butter is a healthy weight loss breakfast combination. Adding starchy carbs to a breakfast of eggs and vegetables with butter, is a different story. That creates a big blood glucose increase and is a weight-gain combination.

Bacon

Bacon also creates very little blood glucose and promotes weight loss as long as it is eaten alone or with eggs or vegetables.

I'm sure this is going to be one of your biggest surprises. It took me decades to figure out why sometimes bacon seemed to have negligible impact on my blood sugar and sometimes it seemed to have a lot of impact. I finally figured out what created the discrepancy.

After thousands of blood sugar tests, I stumbled upon the answer. About 10 years ago I started periodically eating breakfasts with just bacon and eggs or sausage and eggs—no potatoes, no pancakes, no toast. I was stunned at how little impact bacon or sausage with eggs had on my blood glucose and weight. Because those breakfasts created so much less glucose, my need for insulin went way down and I started losing weight without even trying.

Since then I have learned that I can add almost any vegetable—with butter—to that combination of bacon and/or eggs and weight loss will result.

Compare the bacon graph to the single piece of wheat toast with and without butter (Graphs 19 and 20). That comparison provides a good example of the relative contribution to your weight of toast vs. bacon.

Now few people eat bacon alone, although doing so is a good weight loss action. Following this section on protein and fat, you'll find a section titled, "Good Meals, Bad meals," which will show you which *combinations* of foods will trigger high blood sugar and weight gain and which will trigger lower blood sugars and weight loss.

Impact of Glucose Control Eating© on Cholesterol Levels, Circulatory Health, and Heart Health

So if fat's not the problem and starchy carbs are, how about heart health, circulatory health, and cholesterol? As I evolved into applying my Glucose Control Diet© to my eating habits, I was concerned about those issues too—for a while.

But over my years of evolution to my Glucose Control Eating©, my good cholesterol (HDL) increased significantly and my bad cholesterol

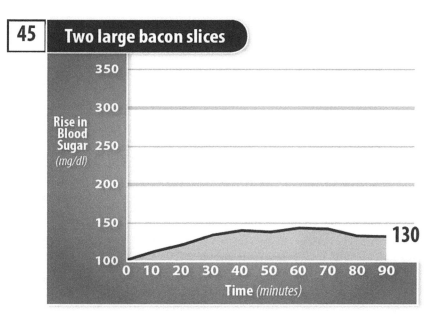

45 **Two large bacon slices**

Total Calories – 86

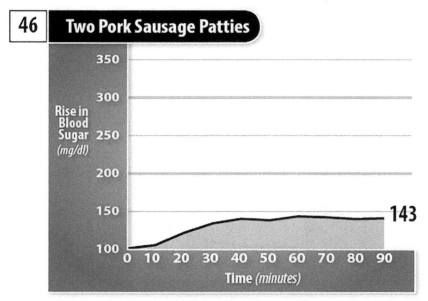

46 **Two Pork Sausage Patties**

Total Calories – 290

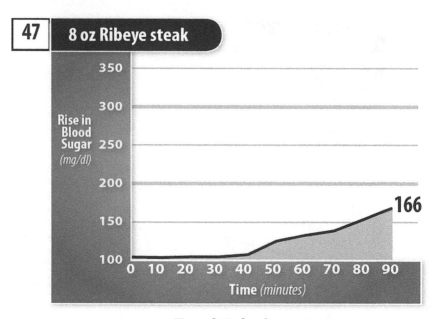

47 | **8 oz Ribeye steak**

Total Calories – 480

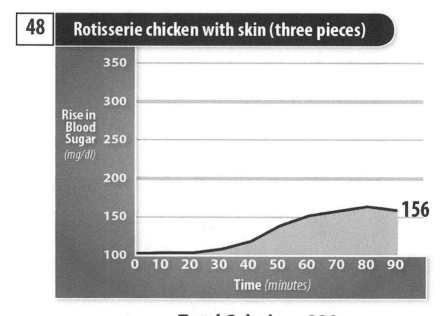

48 | **Rotisserie chicken with skin (three pieces)**

Total Calories – 330

(LDL) decreased. The result is the healthiest ratio of good to bad cholesterol my doctor has seen.

One of the best measures of circulatory health is in the tiny capillaries of your eyes. They are the only visible portion of your circulatory system and damage to those capillaries are a result of circulation problems and a major cause of vision problems. If their circulation is good, you can be comfortable that the rest of your circulatory system is also good.

Here's what my ophthalmologist, who checks my eyes every few years said, "I have never seen anyone with Type 1 diabetes without any evidence of eye damage after a few decades, let alone 50 years after diagnosis."

Regarding my heart health, my doctor of more than 30 years decided two years ago that I should have a complete heart checkup by a cardiologist. Even though by all indications I was healthy, I *was* 75 years old and had never had a complete heart work-up. She scheduled one and I passed with all good news.

But don't just rely on my good health with this diet. In the next chapter, I'll share the evolving medical research on the cause and measurement of cholesterol and the role of fat in heart and circulatory health.

Rib-eye steak and rotisserie chicken are two more examples of the low blood glucose impact of protein and fat if not combined with starchy carbs or sweet carbs. Also notice how many calories both the steak and the chicken have and how little impact they will have on your weight—the shaded area—*if you don't have starchy or sweet carbs in the same meal.* The skin of the rotisserie chicken, unlike breading on some chicken, is not a problem. Eating these two foods along with vegetables with or without butter and maybe a little fruit is a great weight-loss combination. You'll see more graphs illustrating these foods in combinations in the "Good Meals, Bad Meals" section of graphs coming up.

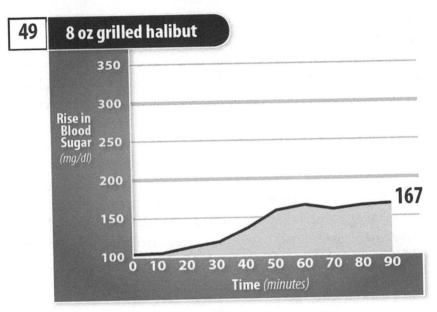

49 **8 oz grilled halibut**

Total Calories – 249

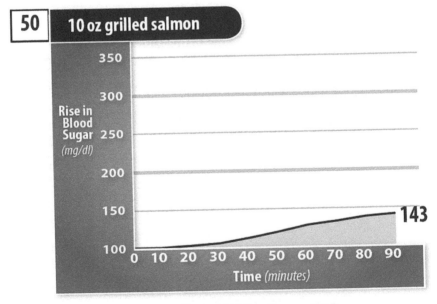

50 **10 oz grilled salmon**

Total Calories – 402

Halibut and Salmon

Both of these cold-water fish are excellent choices to keep blood glucose down and lose weight. In the next group of graphs for "Good Meals, Bad Meals" you'll see how meals with these two fish choices plus cod can contribute to lowering blood glucose and losing weight when combined with other protein, vegetables, and butter or fat-based sauce.

Also note that the piece of salmon is big. A piece ½ that size would have half the impact and would be a great weight-loss meal if not combined with starchy carbs or followed by a sweet dessert.

In terms of general health, it's hard to beat salmon. Consensus agreement among researchers is that the omega-3 fats in salmon improve cholesterol ratios, reduce triglycerides, and generally improve heart and circulatory health.

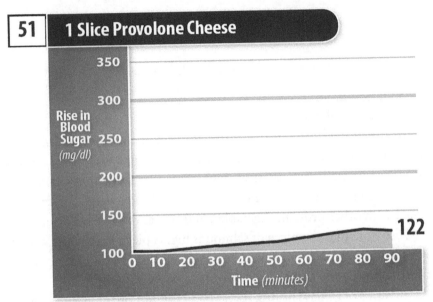

51 — 1 Slice Provolone Cheese

Rise in Blood Sugar *(mg/dl)*

122

Time *(minutes)*

Total Calories – 100

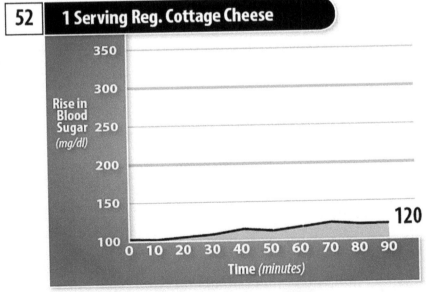

52 — 1 Serving Reg. Cottage Cheese

Rise in Blood Sugar *(mg/dl)*

120

Time *(minutes)*

Total Calories – 222

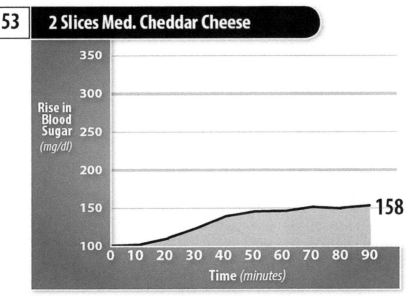

53 **2 Slices Med. Cheddar Cheese**

Total Calories – 200

Cheeses

Most cheese has little impact on blood sugar and weight. They provide a good snack or addition to a meal. Notice the small impact of cottage cheese despite the relatively high calories. I periodically put a small amount of cheddar cheese on a Dixie Ultra paper plate so it won't stick and put it in the microwave for 30 seconds. Cheese has that great quality of tasting a lot better when melted. I smile when I tell an audience that a toasted cheese sandwich without the toast is a healthy snack.

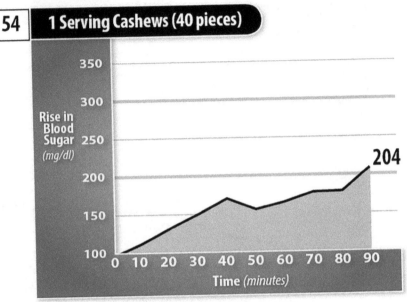

54 | **1 Serving Cashews (40 pieces)**

Rise in Blood Sugar (*mg/dl*)

350
300
250
200
150
100

204

Time (*minutes*)
0 10 20 30 40 50 60 70 80 90

Total Calories – 157

Cashews and Almonds

As you can see by this graph of cashews, they don't raise blood glucose by much or quickly but they are not a free ride. This reflects the impact of 40 cashews which the label says is a "serving." That's too much as a snack. I recommend half that many as a better snack size, and 20 cashews would raise my blood glucose by only half that much. Shaved almonds baked on a flat pan and salted also make a good-tasting and healthy snack.

I've lately become a great fan of pistachios. Looking at the 160 calories per serving makes them seem like a weight-adding snack. It's not the case. Pistachios create both a slow and small rise in blood glucose and you have to work to eat them one at a time. They have little impact on your blood glucose or weight. Don't buy the shelled pistachios as a snack. It's too easy to eat them a handful at a time. If you're looking for something to snack on while you're watching tv, pistachios are good to eat one at a time. My personal favorite as a healthy snack is the Wonderful Pistachios® brand.

Good Meals, Bad Meals

Generally, we don't eat foods individually; we usually combine them and create meals. You now know that sweet carbs and starchy carbs cause big rises in blood sugar and are big contributors to weight gain. Now you will see what happens when you combine those foods with good individual weight-loss foods such as protein, vegetables, or fat. In the following groups of meals, pay close attention to which of the meals have starchy carbs in them and which do not, then note their comparative impacts on blood sugar and therefore on weight gain. It's also important to recall that if you add a sweet to the meal—for example a soft drink—or if you follow a meal with a dessert, it will dramatically increase the glucose creation and weight increase of that whole meal.I realize that having vegetables with eggs for breakfast is a huge shift in eating lifestyles for most Americans. But if you really care about lowering blood sugar, losing weight, and living a longer, healthier life, breakfast is a good *place* to start; replacing toast, pancakes, waffles, or biscuits with vegetables is a good *way* to start. Compare these breakfast graphs (55–60) to the next four breakfast graphs (61–64), which all have some starchy carbs in them. That should provide some motivation to eliminate starchy carbs and include vegetable carbs in your breakfasts, plus you really do have a wide variety of vegetables from which to choose.

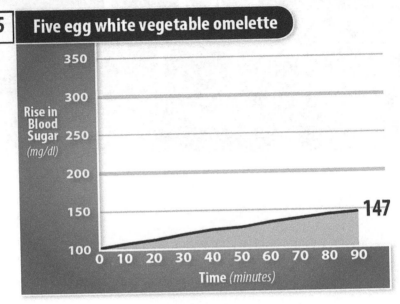

55 **Five egg white vegetable omelette**

Total Calories – 110

Once again, these graphs show that the type of food you eat is much more important than the calories in determining blood glucose increases and weight gain.

A vegetable omelet is one of the best weight-loss breakfasts you can eat. It does not have to be egg whites—it can be eggs with yolks. The yolks will add only about 4 mg/dl to this graph. This breakfast is just the omelet, but it changes dramatically if you add toast, bagels, muffins, or fruit juice.

Black coffee will have no impact on blood glucose and will not neutralize the benefit of this great breakfast. A little cream—not all the high-caloric cream flavors that are so prevalent—and ½ teaspoon of sugar is not a big deal in terms of impact on weight. The lactose in the cream and the eight calories of sugar contribute just slightly to weight in combination with the fat, protein, and vegetables in the omelet.

I don't recommend or use artificial sweeteners. Much better to get accustomed to drinking unsweetened coffee rather than placating and sustaining your desire for a sweet taste. Give coffee without any sweetener a try for a month. You'll soon find it very natural. These two

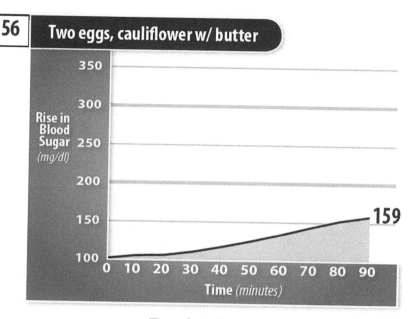

56 Two eggs, cauliflower w/ butter

Total Calories – 230

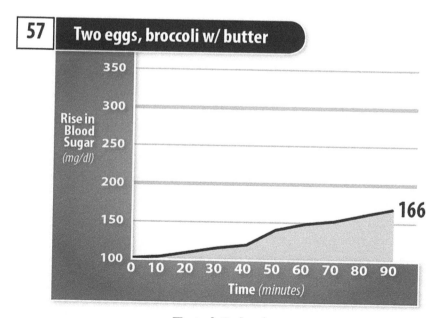

57 Two eggs, broccoli w/ butter

Total Calories – 233

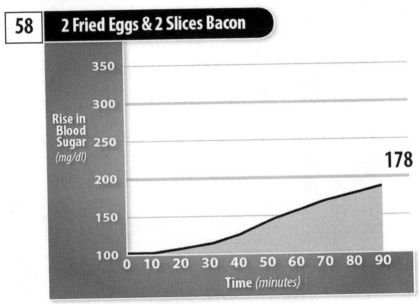

| 58 | 2 Fried Eggs & 2 Slices Bacon |

Total Calories – 266

breakfasts with eggs and vegetables are healthy, good-tasting, and big weight-loss breakfasts. I simply boil or steam the vegetables, but you can be as creative as you want cooking them. Be generous with the butter. The additional benefit of the butter is not being hungry again for four or five hours.

These next three graphs show heavier protein, bigger breakfasts for folks who will be having a more vigorous day at work or workouts. These breakfasts are good for people who want to trim weight but not give up strength.

59 **3 Fried Eggs, Ground Sirloin, Tomato Slices**

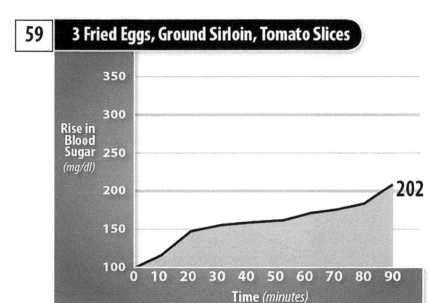

Total Calories – 502

60 **2 Fried Eggs & 10 oz Ground Beef**

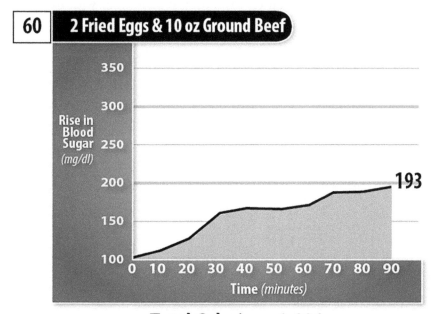

Total Calories – 1,121

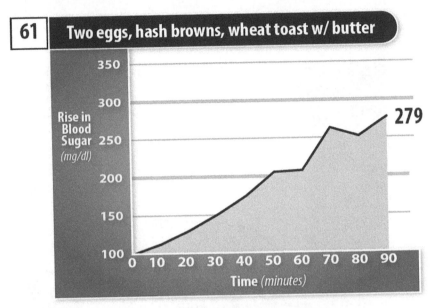

61 Two eggs, hash browns, wheat toast w/ butter

Rise in Blood Sugar (mg/dl)

350
300
279
250
200
150
100

0 10 20 30 40 50 60 70 80 90

Time *(minutes)*

Total Calories – 742

Four of these *weight-gain* breakfasts have starchy carbs added to the protein and fat. One graph (62) is mostly starchy carbs with fruit and skim milk added.

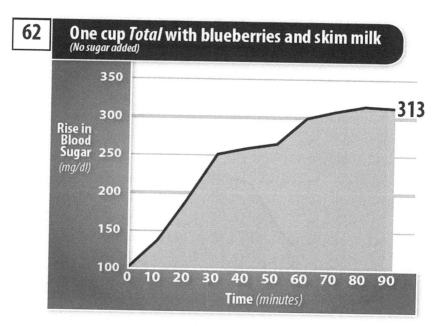

62 One cup *Total* with blueberries and skim milk
(No sugar added)

Total Calories – 232

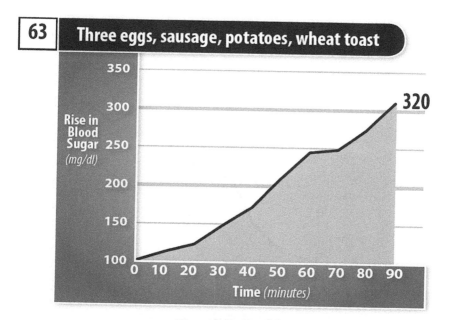

63 Three eggs, sausage, potatoes, wheat toast

Total Calories – 687

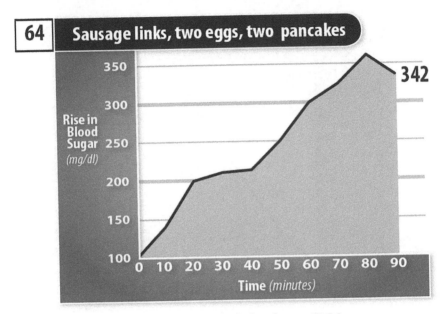

64 Sausage links, two eggs, two pancakes

342

Total Calories – 761

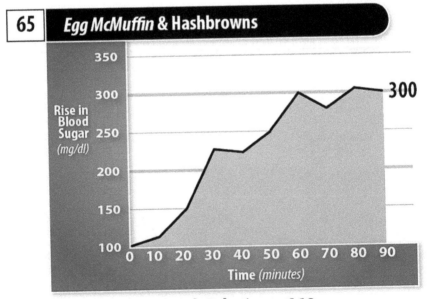

65 *Egg McMuffin* & Hashbrowns

300

Total Calories – 460

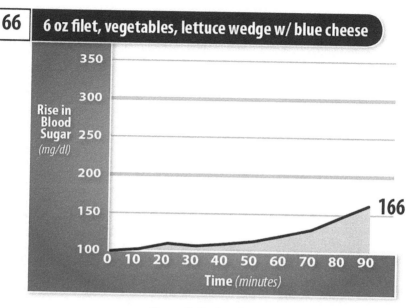

66 6 oz filet, vegetables, lettuce wedge w/ blue cheese

Total Calories – 692

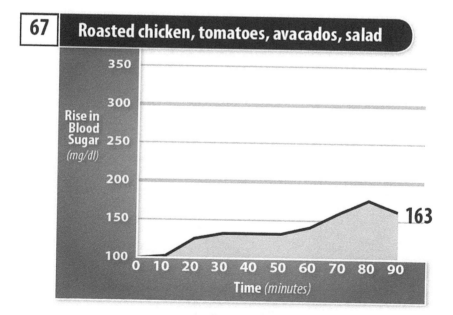

67 Roasted chicken, tomatoes, avacados, salad

Total Calories – 413

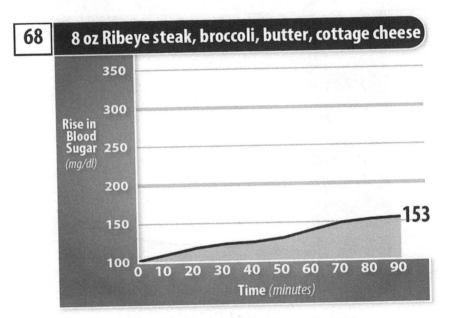

68 | **8 oz Ribeye steak, broccoli, butter, cottage cheese**

Total Calories – 1,120

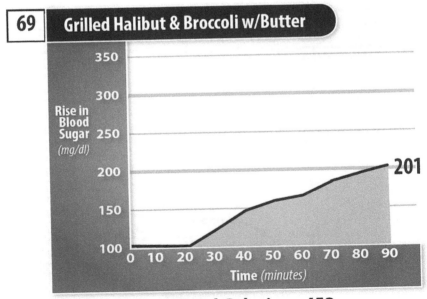

69 | **Grilled Halibut & Broccoli w/Butter**

Total Calories – 453

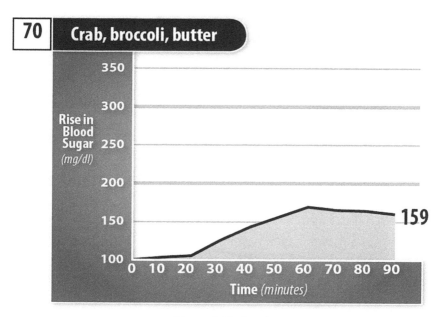

Total Calories – 396

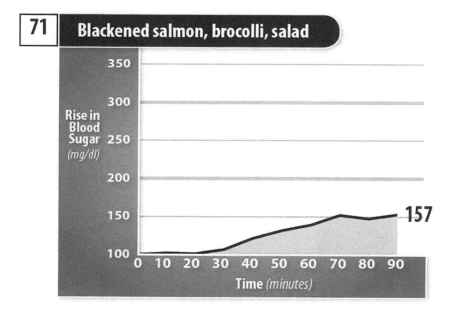

Total Calories – 336

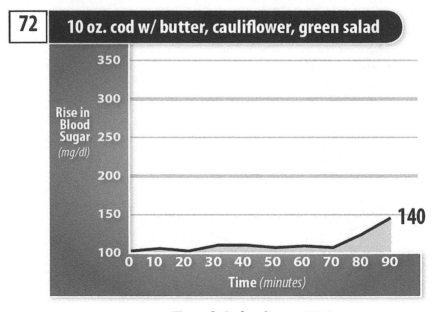

Total Calories – 291

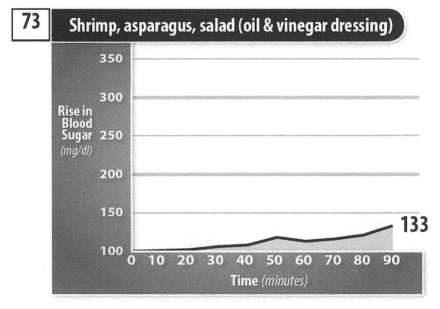

Total Calories – 140

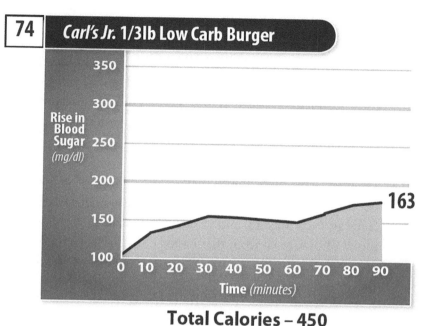

74 *Carl's Jr.* **1/3lb Low Carb Burger**

Rise in Blood Sugar *(mg/dl)*

163

Time *(minutes)*

Total Calories – 450

The preceding group of nine graphs illustrates three major points of Glucose Control Eating©:

1. Fat when combined with protein and vegetables is an excellent combination to promote the loss of weight and body fat.

2. All these meals have small impacts on blood glucose and therefore promote weight loss.

3. Adding more fat to a meal that does not include starchy carbs or sweet carbs will have little impact on blood glucose and makes a good weight-loss-promoting meal. Compare the 6 oz. filet steak to the 8 oz. rib-eye steak. The rib-eye has more fat than the lower-fat filet; but both have a similar small impact on blood glucose and therefore on weight.

4. This group of graphs also demonstrates the importance of seafood in Glucose Control Eating©. Salmon, crab, halibut, cod, and shrimp are all excellent choices for weight loss. It makes no difference whether they're baked, grilled, sautéed, fried, steamed, or boiled as long as you don't add breading to the seafood. You can freely add butter and fat-based sauces, but not breading.

5. The final point these graphs make is the significant weight-loss benefit of roasted chicken. I tested the roasted chicken from Safeway, Fred Meyer's, and Costco. The graph shows three pieces of dark meat from the roasted chicken. In each case the tests include the skin. Graph 67 also includes more fat from the avocado and from the blue cheese dressing on the salad.

None of the preceding weight-loss meals include starchy carbs or sweet carbs, and none are followed by a dessert. Now compare these graphs with the next four high-blood-sugar, weight-gain dinners.

These graphs show what happens when you add starchy carbs to meals high in protein and fat and when you eat meals primarily consisting of starchy carbs.

Once again, compare the size of the shaded area of the weight-loss dinners to the size of the gray area of the weight-gain dinners. Think of that gray area as added body fat. You don't have to count calories you just need to visualize the gray areas.

Eat meals like the weight-loss dinners—protein, fat, and vegetables with perhaps a little fruit added—and you will see and feel your body fat melting away.

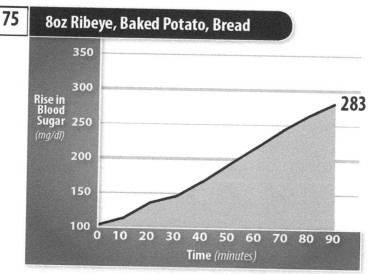

75 **8oz Ribeye, Baked Potato, Bread**

Total Calories – 618

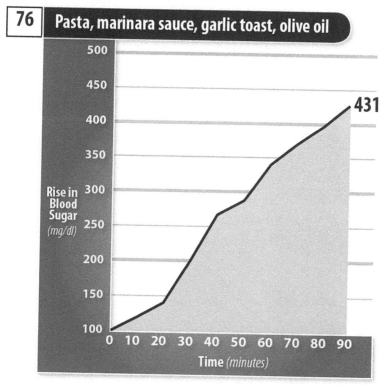

76 **Pasta, marinara sauce, garlic toast, olive oil**

Total Calories – 780

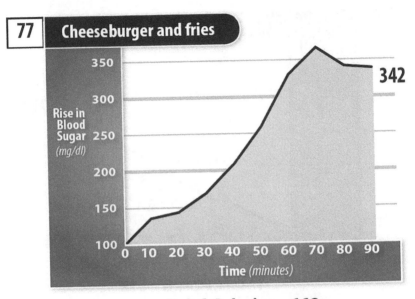

Total Calories – 668

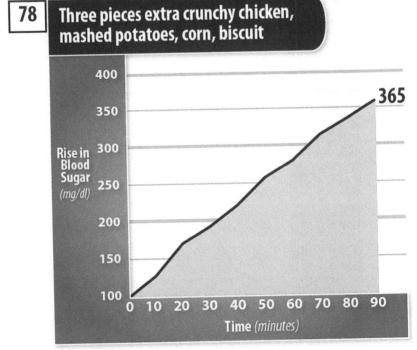

Total Calories – 1,600

Yogurt

I don't eat much yogurt but my testing of original vs. non-fat yogurt further illustrates my conclusions that "it's not fat that makes people fat. It's starchy and sweet carbohydrates." Low-fat or no-fat yogurts always list fewer calories and less fat than original or traditional yogurts. That must mean that low-fat or no-fat yogurts will create less blood glucose increase and less weight gain. Right? No. Wrong!

Why do the graphs show that original yogurt will create less glucose and promote weight loss better than no-fat and low-fat varieties that have fewer calories?

It's because the no-fat and low-fat varieties have more sweet or starchy carbs to compensate for the taste given up by taking out the fat. If they take out the 9-calorie-per-gram fat and replace it with 5-calorie-per-gram carbs, the calories will go down. But the issue is not the number of calories, it's the type of food. These graphs illustrate beautifully that more sweet and starchy carbs and less fat is the problem. Fewer carbs and more fat are the solutions. Give up that chalky, bad-tasting, no-fat yogurt and enjoy the better-tasting original or traditional yogurt—if you can find it among the densely packed shelves of low-fat yogurt.

You'll also see in the last two graphs that fruit-flavored or fruit-on-the-bottom yogurts are big contributors to weight gain.

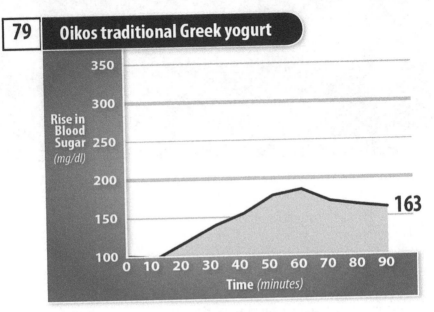

79 Oikos traditional Greek yogurt

163

Total Calories – 63

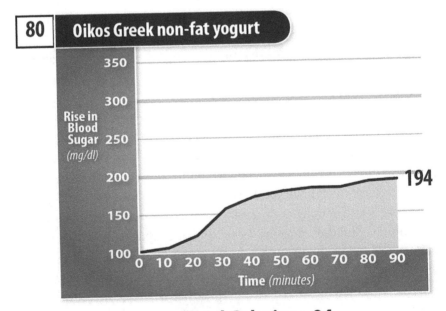

80 Oikos Greek non-fat yogurt

194

Total Calories – 94

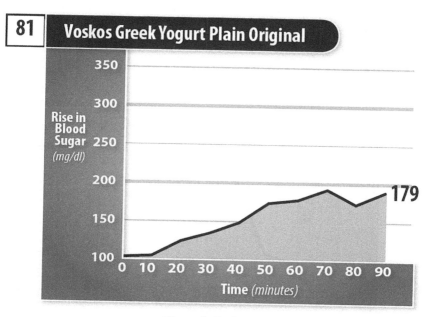

81 **Voskos Greek Yogurt Plain Original**

Total Calories –79

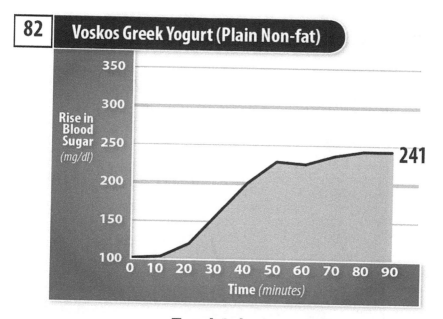

82 **Voskos Greek Yogurt (Plain Non-fat)**

Total Calories – 141

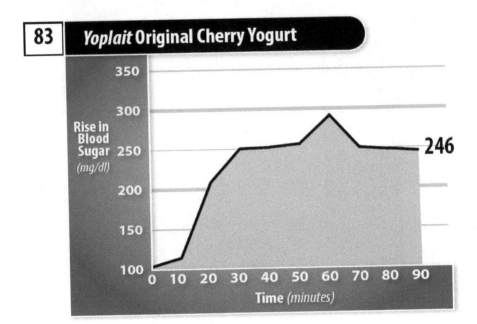

83 *Yoplait* Original Cherry Yogurt

Rise in Blood Sugar *(mg/dl)*

246

Time *(minutes)*

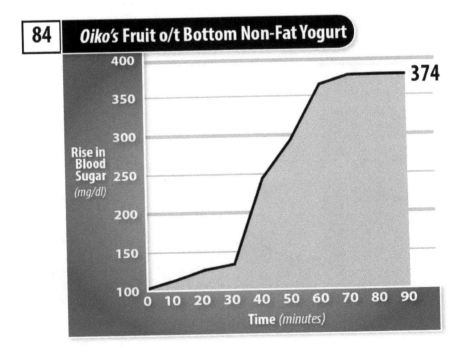

84 *Oiko's* Fruit o/t Bottom Non-Fat Yogurt

Rise in Blood Sugar *(mg/dl)*

374

Time *(minutes)*

Chapter 6

A Brief Review of Actions to Take and What Others Say About the Role of Fat in a Healthy Eating

In this chapter, I explain how the results of my tests and my experiences measuring my own blood glucose are coincidentally gaining support in the research and medical communities. I'll also be referring you to medical researchers and doctors who argue convincingly that it's not fat that creates high cholesterol and high triglyceride levels, which are the big precursors of circulatory and heart problems. It's sweet carbs and starchy carbs that cause those problems.

First—A Review

Friends and Foes of Weight Loss

Protein and Vegetable Carbs—Your good Friends
Fruit Carbs—Your mostly good Friends
Fats—Your conditional friends
Starchy Carbs and Sweet Carbs—Your Foes

Now that you've had a chance to study the graphs, let's **review** the key actions of Glucose Control Eating©.

Eliminate or Dramatically Minimize Sweet Carbohydrates— Except for Very Special Occasions
They are your weight-loss foes

You now know this category of foods enters your bloodstream very quickly and causes large and fast increases in blood glucose and therefore weight. Most sweet carbohydrates will show up in blood glucose tests in two or three minutes.

The simple sugars with no fat mixed in are the quickest to enter the bloodstream and you now know that is bad. Sugared soft drinks, Skittles, Starbursts, jelly beans and other candies that are simple sugars fall into this category. Baked desserts such as cakes and pies usually have some fat in them, as do chocolate candy bars and ice cream. As you now know, fat enters your bloodstream more slowly, so when fat mixes with sweet carbohydrates in your stomach, the combination creates a bigger but somewhat slower increase in blood glucose than just sugared sweets or drinks. However, the fat, hitching a ride with the sweets, results in a big rise in blood sugar and is a major contributor to weight.

Minimize Starchy Carbohydrates
They Are Your Weight-Loss Foes Too

You've seen from the graphs that starchy carbs are also a category of carbohydrates that raise your blood sugar very quickly and result in an increase as great as that of sweet carbs.

Although most people realize that sweets are big contributors to weight gain and to Type 2 diabetes, very few realize how much starchy carbs contribute to our national obesity and to our Type 2 diabetes epidemic. Starchy carbs may be even bigger contributors to our overweight problem because people in general eat a larger volume of starchy carbs than of sweet carbs.

A big step you can take to lower your blood sugars and reduce your weight is to dramatically minimize your consumption of starchy and sweet carbohydrates.

How does the Beef Industry Makes Cows
As Fat As Possible As Fast As Possible?

As I said in the lead-in to this section, fats are not the villains they are made out to be. For years we have read over and over about losing weight with low-fat diets. We have read about low-fat this and low-fat that. Who argued? It seemed so reasonable. If you don't want to get fat then don't eat fat. Simple, right?

Think about this for a minute—if eating fat makes people fat, one would think it would hold true for animals too. After all, enough similarities exist between mice and humans that mice are continually being tested by scientists to see how humans might react to the same food, medications, or environmental situations.

The beef industry has an incentive to make its cows as fat as possible as fast as possible. Do they feed their cows fat? No!

Over the last 80 years in America, the beef industry has learned how to make cows *as fat as possible as fast as possible.* How do they do it? They grow their cattle in feedlots on a diet of feed consisting primarily of corn and grains…and remember I said corn was one of the two vegetables that act like starchy carbs. I would call this feed stock, starchy carbohydrates for cows.

How often have you heard or read the term "pure corn-fed beef?" Corn- and grain-dominated feed makes cows fat quickly and gives beef a juicier, fattier texture—and likely a better taste. This is great for the beef industry and for all of us who enjoy a tasty, juicy steak periodically. But is this what you want for yourself—*to get as fat as possible as fast as possible?*

The next time you're getting ready to eat a nice rib-eye steak, remind yourself that the cow that nicely marbled steak came from ate not one ounce of fat.

What Others Say

In Dr. William Davis's excellent book, *Wheat Belly,* (Rodale, 2011), Dr. Davis came to conclusions very similar to the conclusions I've come to. He first introduces the problem with what I call starchy carbs with the following headline on the back cover of his book, "DID YOU KNOW THAT EATING TWO SLICES OF WHOLE WHEAT BREAD CAN INCREASE BLOOD SUGAR MORE THAN TWO TABLESPOONS OF PURE SUGAR CAN?"

Early in his book he describes what he calls "wheat belly."

> A wheat belly represents the accumulation of fat that results from years of consuming goods that trigger insulin, the hormone of fat storage. While some people store fat in their buttocks and thighs, most people collect ungainly fat around the middle.

Dr. Davis also talks about the lethargy and drowsiness that results from eating wheat-based foods for breakfast instead of protein and fat. He states, "I couldn't help but notice that on the days when I'd eat toast, waffles, or bagels for breakfast, I'd stumble through several hours of sleepiness and lethargy. But eat a three-egg omelet with cheese and I feel fine."

In his book, he also refers to the success he has had with his patients who replaced wheat-based foods with other, healthier whole foods.

> After three months, my patients returned to have more blood work done. As I had anticipated, with only rare exceptions, blood sugar (glucose) had indeed often dropped from diabetic range (126 mg/dl or greater) to normal. Yes, diabetics became nondiabetics. That's right: Diabetes in many cases can be cured—not simply managed—by removal of carbohydrates, especially wheat from the diet. Many of my patients lost twenty, thirty, even forty pounds.

Two items in that quote deserve a response. First, when he talks about diabetics becoming nondiabetics, I'm sure he is referring to Type 2 diabetics. Second, I do not advocate the removal of all carbohydrates from a diet. I advocate dramatically limiting sweet carbohydrates and

---

AUTHOR'S NOTE:
The weight loss and curing of diabetes by eating eggs and other protein for breakfast is what my readers have experienced also.

starchy carbohydrates; protein, fat, and vegetable carbohydrates do not need to be limited at all and fruit carbohydrates just need to be moderately limited.

Eat Moderate Amounts of Fruit Carbs
Most Fruit Carbs Are Okay.
Fruit carbs vary quite a bit, but the graphs should have helped you understand their general impact. The basic message regarding fruit carbohydrates is that they will raise blood sugar a little more than veggie carbs, protein, and fat but way less than sweet or starchy carbs. Fruits include many vitamins and water-soluble fibers that are important to general good health.

Including fruits as part of your eating lifestyle is okay. However, in my experience fruits such as pineapples, peaches, bananas, and strawberries will raise blood sugar fairly fast and need to be eaten in moderation in order to maintain lower blood glucose and lose weight.

Fruit juices are a different story. They are problematic in causing fast and big weight gains.

In many cases, a large glass of apple juice, orange juice, or pineapple juice for breakfast will raise your blood sugar more and put on more weight than all the rest of your breakfast combined, and it gets into your bloodstream much faster than you can use it, so it gets stored in and around your body.

An Associated Press article from the December 11, 2011 edition of the *Honolulu Star* newspaper supports what I learned from my testing.

> Apple juice is far from nutritious. Nutrition experts say apple juice's real danger is to waistlines and children's teeth. Apple juice has few natural nutrients, lots of calories, and in some cases, more sugar than soda. It trains a child to like sweet things, displaces better beverages and foods, and adds to the obesity problem.

Freely Eat Veggie Carbohydrates
They Are Your Weight-loss Friends.

As you learned from the graphs, vegetable carbs are an excellent group of foods for lowering blood glucose and losing weight. Not only do these foods have lots of nutrients but they also enter your bloodstream more slowly than the previous three categories. This means that you can burn the calories from these carbohydrates before they get stored as glycogen in your liver or as fat around your body. These are the foods your mom told you to eat. She was right. They include most vegetables except the starchy ones I mentioned earlier—corn and potatoes.

"Eat Produce, Live Longer" was the headline of a March 17, 2017 story in *The Week* magazine. The story went on to explain.

> After analyzing 95 studies on diet and well-being, researchers from the Imperial College London have concluded that we should be aiming to eat 10 portions of fruit and vegetables a day, rather than the five portions recommended by the World Health Organization. They found that the daily consumption of 28 ounces of fresh produce was associated with a 33 percent reduced risk of stroke, a 13 percent drop in cancer risk, and a 33 percent lower risk for premature death.

To lose weight, I recommend no more than two servings of fruit a day.

Freely Eat Proteins
They Are Your Friends Too.

Proteins have gone in and out of favor many times in the past 60 years. From my experience over the past 35 years of blood glucose testing, I've made protein a very significant part of my diet to keep my blood sugars in control and weight down. While protein has little effect on blood glucose, it has a noticeably positive effect on my muscle growth when I match increased protein with strength training.

As you could tell from the graphs, protein will cause neither a quick nor a significant rise in blood glucose. Consequently, I freely eat large quantities of protein with a barely measurable effect on my blood glucose.

Here's a review of protein that you can eat often and freely without weight gain: salmon, halibut, cod, trout, shrimp, scallops, chicken and turkey (with skin but without breading), Cornish game hen, beef (including corned beef and cabbage—a great weight-loss meal) ham, and pork.

My core protein food is Wild Alaska salmon. I eat it two or three times a week in the summer and maybe once a week in the winter. It is an almost perfect food. With minimal impact on my blood sugar, it is absorbed slowly so the small amount of glucose it creates is burned as fast as it goes into the bloodstream and doesn't get stored as fat.

Salmon is not only high in protein but also high in omega-3 fatty acids (which all my reading indicates is a good fat). Salmon is also a good source of vitamin D. All that and it tastes great too. Just don't overcook it.

Eat Fat Freely
Fat Promotes Weight Loss when Eaten Alone or Combined with Vegetables and/or Proteins Such As Fish or Meat.
Fat Promotes Weight Gain When Eaten with Starchy Carbs in the Same Meal or When Followed by a Sweet Dessert.

I spend more time talking about fat in this book than about any other of the food groups because my research and conclusions are significantly different from what our Government through the Department of Agriculture has told us for nearly two generations.

The impact of fats has been the biggest surprise —maybe revelation is a better word—to me over my years of testing. You can see from the graphs in the previous chapter that adding butter to vegetables has almost no blood sugar impact, that bacon alone has minimal impact, that eggs with the yolk have almost no blood sugar impact.

I probably add more butter to my foods than 90 percent of Americans, and have for 30 years, but I eat very few baked desserts, so I don't get all the butter or other fats that are combined with starchy and sweet carbs in those foods. And I rarely eat butter on starchy carbs like breads, biscuits, muffins, bagels and so forth.

Because most of my butter is used on vegetables, eggs, and fish, my blood profile and cholesterol ratios of good cholesterol (HDL) to bad cholesterol (LDL) are, in the words of my doctor, the best she has ever seen in her extensive practice.

Many Researchers Are Now Promoting Fat as A Healthy Part of a Diet.

What Others Say!

On June 23, 2014, *Time Magazine's* cover headlined the words **"Eat Butter."** The subhead declared **"Scientists labeled fat the enemy. Why they were wrong."**

The New York Times on February 19, 2015 said "…major health groups like the American Heart Association in recent years have backed away from dietary cholesterol restrictions."

Runner's World magazine in their January/February 2015 edition in a story titled "Eat Fat, Be Fit" led the story as follows:

> Runners like to follow the rules. And for decades, nutrition rules put a strict limit on saturated fat. After all, as far back as the 1960s, experts have decreed that eating foods high in saturated fat such as eggs, red meat, and full-fat dairy, will increase your risk of heart disease. So runners took heed, all but banishing those foods from their diets.
>
> But a string of news-making studies has flipped that idea on its head. One of those headline-catchers published in the Annals of Internal Medicine early last year, reviewed 76 existing studies and found no association between saturated fat and heart disease. The new emerging thought (is): "Saturated fat may not be the demon that it was made out to be," says Jeff Volek, Ph.D., R.D., associate professor in the department of kinesiology at the University of Connecticut.

I've become more aligned in my thinking with the growing number of researchers and doctors who no longer believe fat is the villain it has been made out to be.

The best-known advocate for a general low-carbohydrate diet is Dr. Robert Atkins, who in 2002 wrote Dr. Atkins New Diet Revolution.

Some of his conclusions were different from mine. He didn't break down carbohydrates into the categories that I believe are so important to weight loss and Type 2 diabetes reversal.

A few years ago, I saw a clip from an interview Dr. Atkins had many years before with Barbara Walters. In this interview she said to him, "Are you telling me that I can eat as much fat as I want and won't gain weight?" He simply and emphatically said, "Yes, if you don't eat that fat with carbohydrates." That means—according to Dr. Atkins— fat is a good weight loss food only if you eat it solely with protein. That is a very limiting use of butter, for example.

My Research and Conclusions Are Somewhat Different

My conclusions are different but important. Fat is a good weight-loss food when eaten with protein *and veggie carbs* in a meal. You can put all the butter you want on the vegetables— except for corn and potatoes—and it will contribute almost nothing to blood glucose or weight gain.

That is, in fact, a very significant difference because it shows that you can eat vegetable carbohydrates with butter or other fat and it will have very little impact on your weight. But if you eat butter, for example, with bread, rice, pasta, or spaghetti, or if you follow a meal with a dessert (sweet carbs), then that butter will contribute to weight gain.

You will find that by putting butter liberally on vegetables as well as crab, lobster, salmon, halibut, cod, trout, catfish, pollock, shrimp, and other seafood, you will eat more vegetables and more fish—all great contributors to weight-loss and good health.

Doctor Eric Westman, Director of the Duke University Lifestyle Medicine Clinic

Dr. Eric Westman, director of the Duke Lifestyle Medicine Clinic and one of the authors of *A New Atkins for a New You*, has been studying low-carbohydrate diets for 12 years and says, "…when it comes to protein and fat, eat as much as you want. You don't have to use portion control. Your hunger will go down when you start eating this way—all you have to do is stop eating when you're full." He also says, "Say goodbye to pasta, rice, bread, and corn."

My testing generally supports what Dr. Westman is saying but Glucose Control Eating© also includes vegetables (veggie carbs) as a food group you can eat freely with butter with no weight gain.

Gary Taubes's Book, *Why We Get Fat—And What to Do About It.*
In an article by Lisa Davis in the February 11, 2011 issue of *Reader's Digest,* she writes about Gary Taubes's book, *Why We Get Fat—And What to Do About It.*

Taubes is an award-winning science journalist.

Davis writes,

> "If obesity researchers are so smart, why are we so large? After all, public health authorities have been hammering home a very simple message for the past 40 years. If you don't want to be fat, cut the fat from your diet. And in those years, obesity rates have gone from 13 percent to 22 percent to—in the last national survey—33 percent."

> Taubes thinks he knows why: "Obesity experts have gotten things just about completely backward. If you look carefully at the research, he says, fat isn't the enemy; easily digested carbohydrates are. The very foods that we've been sold as diet staples—fat-free yogurt, plain baked potatoes—hold the butter—and plain pasta—hold the olive oil, sauce, and cheese—actually reset our physiology to make us pack on the pounds. And the foods that we've been told to shun— steak, burgers, cheese, even the sour cream so carefully scraped from that potato—can help us finally lose the weight and keep our hearts healthy."

Taubes continues with his message under the heading "High Fat is Better for Your Heart." Regarding the low-carb, high-fat diet he says, "Your HDL [the good cholesterol] goes up, which is the most meaningful number in terms of heart health. Not only does your cholesterol profile get better, your insulin goes down, your insulin resistance goes away, and your blood pressure goes down."

He continues, "The low-fat diet that people have been eating in hopes of protecting their heart is actually bad for their heart."

He argues that diets high in carbohydrates are one of the fundamental reasons that we now have obesity and diabetes epidemics. I would add to that and say, it's diets high in starchy carbohydrates and sweet carbohydrates that have been one of the biggest causes of our Type 2 diabetes and obesity epidemic.

In 2007, Taubes published _Good Calories, Bad Calories: Challenging the Conventional Wisdom on Diet, Weight Control and Disease_, a book that led the _New York Times_ to assert that "Gary Taubes is a brave and bold science journalist" who shows that "much of what is believed about nutrition and health is based on the flimsiest evidence."

Taubes's message: Political pressure and sloppy science over the last 50 years have skewed research to make it seem that dietary fat and cholesterol are the main causes of obesity and heart disease, but there are, in fact, few or no objective data to support that hypothesis.

A more careful look (Taubes researched his book for five years; its 450 pages include 60 pages of footnotes) reveals that the real obesity-epidemic drivers are increased consumption of refined carbohydrates, mainly sugar and white flour.

Bottom line: Taubes says, "Carbohydrates are driving insulin, and insulin is driving fat deposition." When it comes to accumulating fat, carbohydrates are indeed "bad calories," as they are the only ones that boost insulin and make fat accumulation possible.

My 40 years of blood glucose tests show that the villains are _sweet_ and starchy carbs—not vegetable carbs, fat, protein, or most fruit carbs.

What's the scientific weight-loss solution? Taubes asserted that since the fewer carbohydrates we eat, the leaner we will be, our diets should emphasize meat, fish, fowl, cheese, butter, eggs, and nonstarchy vegetables.

Conversely, we should reduce, or preferably eliminate, bread and other baked goods, potatoes, yams, rice, pasta, cereal grains, corn, sugar (both sucrose and high-fructose corn syrup), ice cream, candy, soft drinks, fruit juices, bananas and other tropical fruits, and beer. Excluding [sweet and starchy]* carbohydrates from the diet, he said, derails the

---

* Author's Parentheses

insulin peak/dip roller coaster, so one is never voraciously hungry, making weight loss and healthy weight maintenance easy.

According to Taubes and supported by my testing, "When you eat this way, the fat just melts off."

"Sugar Tied to Fatal Heart Woes"

On February 5, 2014, the *Anchorage Daily News* ran an Associated Press Article by Lindsey Tanner. The headline was "Sugar tied to fatal heart woes."

The article said the American Centers for Disease Control and Prevention studied more than 30,000 American adults with an average age of 44. Lead author Quanhe Yang called the results sobering and said it's the first nationally representative study to examine the issue.

The article stated,

> Scientists aren't certain exactly how sugar may contribute to deadly heart problems, but it has been shown to increase blood pressure and levels of unhealthy cholesterol and triglycerides, and also may increase signs of inflammation linked with heart disease,' said Rachel Johnson, head of the American Heart Association's nutrition committee and a University of Vermont nutrition professor.

A Good Reference Book on Diabetes

One of the best books I've found on blood sugar control and health is Dr. Bernstein's DIABETES SOLUTION by Richard K. Bernstein, MD. It's very clearly and persuasively written by a doctor who has lived with Type 1 diabetes for "65 years and counting."

AUTHOR'S NOTE:
I think within a few years, this type of research will also identify starchy carbs as contributors to those same heart problems, elevated cholesterol, and triglycerides caused by sugars. This is just one more bit of support for my argument that elevated glucose is a major contributor to these problems. It's not fat— unless of course the fat is accompanied in your meals by sweet or starchy carbs.

Dr. Bernstein uses the words "in theory" when he talks about acquiring more body fat from a fat-free, sweetened dessert than from a "steak nicely marbled with fat." My graphs showed you that it's not just "in theory." It is reality.

The Evolution of Opinions on Fat

These magazines covers are also in Chapter 1, but the evolution of opinions on the role of fat in healthy eating is important enough to include again after you have seen the graphs in chapter 5.

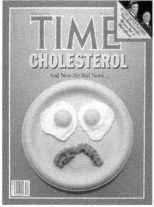

TIME Magazine March 1994

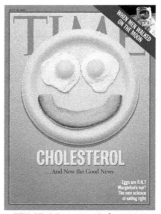

TIME Magazine July 1999

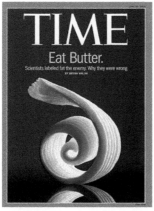

TIME Magazine June 2014*

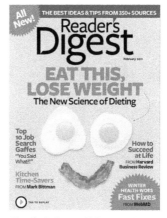

Reader's Digest February 2011

---

* On June 23, 2014, *Time Magazine's* cover headlined the words "Eat Butter." The sub-head declared *"Scientists labeled fat the enemy. Why they were wrong."*

Conclusion

First, remember my previous explanation that the simplest definition of carbs is this: *If a food is not a protein or a fat, then it's a carb.* You now know that *sweets* are carbs, *starchy foods* are carbs, *fruits* are carbs, and *vegetables* are carbs.

To really understand what you should eat and what you shouldn't eat, you must understand that carbs should not be universally condemned or universally praised. Review the graphs, and you'll see that veggie carbs along with protein are a perfect food to load up on and add all the butter you want. Fruit carbs are a little more likely to raise blood glucose but on balance are still good.

To successfully lose weight, you must dramatically reduce starchy carbs and eliminate— or very nearly eliminate—sweet carbs.

In the next chapter, you'll learn how to develop these new eating patterns at breakfast, lunch, dinner, and snacks.

Chapter 7

Developing Your New Eating Habits

Getting Started on Your Glucose Control Eating©

Now that you know what to eat to lose weight, you just need to know how to get started.

Apply what you have learned so far and will learn in the next few chapters, and you will begin losing weight in days. You will feel better, look better, and be on your way to a longer, healthier life.

Breakfast

1. Be Sure to Dilute (or Avoid) Fruit Juices

You saw in chapter 5 how fast and how much orange juice and apple juice raise blood sugar and add to weight.

The pattern you need to start here is to *avoid or dilute juice*. Some people, as I do, have juice only periodically in the morning but many of you may drink juice at different times throughout the day, thinking that it's the healthy thing to do. *It's not.*

The impact on blood glucose and weight counteracts the positive benefit you may get. Though I didn't include pineapple juice in the graphs, it's very similar to orange and apple juice in its impact.

The way to get some benefit from the vitamins that are present in juices is to dilute your juices before you drink them. In the morning, I fill about ¼ of a juice glass with the juice and fill the rest with water. You'll be surprised how easy it is to get used to diluted juices. It won't take long before full-strength orange, apple, cranberry, or even grapefruit juice will feel very thick and very sugary.

The best juice for keeping blood sugar and weight down is V-8 juice. You can choose to dilute it but that's not necessary. I dilute V-8 juice by using a full-size 8 oz. glass—not a juice glass— and putting about ½ glass of V-8 juice in it and filling the rest with sparkling water. It's a very refreshing drink that you will soon become accustomed to.

An Example of Losing More than 20 Pounds Solely by Cutting Back on Orange Juice

The benefit you reap from this change will depend on how much juice you currently drink. If you're a big juice drinker, the benefit will be great. A good example of a huge benefit comes via Barbara Mee, a longtime friend and former special assistant to the late Senator Ted Stevens. Barbara had heard me speak about diabetes. Among the tips I suggested to lower blood sugar and lose weight was to dilute or eliminate certain juices.

Barbara's husband, Vince, worked in street maintenance for the Municipality of Anchorage. His work at that time involved driving snowplows in the winter and driving trucks the rest of the year. Vince was overweight at the time and thinking he was being very conscientious about his health, he would start his day with a big 20-ounce mug of orange juice in his plow.

Soon after Barbara told him about my orange juice suggestion, Vince—coincidentally—had a doctor's appointment. He told the doctor about my advice and the doctor strongly agreed. According to Vince, the doctor told him he needed to lose weight and the first thing he should do was "get off that orange juice." As Vince quoted his doctor, "That's like mainlining sugar." He immediately quit drinking it on the job and cut way back to just a little diluted orange juice for breakfast. Barbara said within months Vince had lost "…25 pounds solely by cutting back on the huge amount of orange juice he drank."

Now both Barbara and Vince are enjoying a well-deserved and active retirement in Florida. They're playing golf together three or four days a week. Vince has never regained the weight he lost after cutting way back on orange juice.

2. Eliminate or Dramatically Reduce Toast, Muffins, and Bagels for Breakfast

For so many years, many health-conscious people thought eating some toast, a bagel with cream cheese or a muffin was a decent, healthy breakfast. *Not so.* In terms of weight gain let's look at these choices.

Toast and English muffins

If you can't eliminate them, at least eat very small portions, like half of a piece of toast or a quarter of a muffin. But if you eat two pieces of toast that's quadruple the starchy carbs. And if you add jelly or jam that's another 30 calories of sweet carbs that will get into your bloodstream so fast that unless you run to work, you won't burn it before it will get stored in the liver as glycogen and then later on your stomach, legs, or hips as fat.

Bagels

Bagels are big. Bagels are starchy. Bagels will send your blood sugar through the roof and make you fat. They will be converted to glucose and enter your bloodstream as glucose faster than you can burn it. Eliminate bagels from your breakfast.

Cinnamon and Sugar vs. Jam or Jelly

If you must have a piece of toast in the morning, do yourself a favor and put a mixture of sugar and cinnamon on it instead of jam or jelly. What— sugar? Yes, cinnamon and sugar. Years ago when I still ate toast for breakfast, I had a feeling that jelly on my toast had a bigger impact on my blood sugar than cinnamon and sugar. I started experimenting with my blood testing and found out it was true.

As an experiment, I put the same amount of cinnamon and sugar that I put on my toast into a teaspoon. It turned about to be ½ teaspoon. Figuring the sugar was about 50% of the mixture, I was putting about ¼ teaspoon of sugar on my toast. At 17 calories per teaspoon of sugar I was adding a little more than 4 calories to my toast; compare that to 32 to 36 calories that jelly added. Some would say it's not a big deal; it only saves about 30 calories a day.

I'd say look at it this way: that simple, small daily action if done daily, would save 210 calories a week, which is the number of calories in one Hershey bar. That means putting jelly or jam on your toast every morning instead of cinnamon and sugar is equivalent to adding 52 candy bars a year to your eating pattern. This is such a good illustration of how making a little change in a daily habit can add up to a meaningful weight loss in a year. Of course, better for your weight loss if you just don't eat toast at all.

3. Eliminate Cereal from Your Breakfast Pattern

Remember when we were kids? We'd wake up and pour ourselves as much cereal as would fit in the bowl, put lots of sugar on it, maybe a banana, and then go out and play for three or four hours. If you're going out after breakfast to play for three or four hours, go ahead and load up on cereal. But if you're not, you must cut back—or eliminate cereal. Look at the graphs one more time and note the impact of cereal on your blood sugar and your weight.

It's the starchy carbohydrate issue. Unless you're going to be very active after breakfast, the cereal will be stored faster than you will burn it and it will trigger storage of the glucose in your liver as glycogen and then around your body as body fat. You're much better off cutting out cereal and eating eggs, some vegetable, and some breakfast meat—if you wish—for your breakfast. The protein and fat in the egg and meat option will go very slowly into your bloodstream and allow you to burn the small amount of glucose that protein and fat create before it ever gets stored.

4. Do Not Eat Sweet Carbohydrates for Breakfast

I'm sure most of you don't do that but if you do eat doughnuts or sweet rolls for breakfast, *stop* for the sake of your blood glucose control, your weight, and your health. Review the charts in chapter 5 and see how much a single medium cherry Danish or a donut will raise blood sugar in just 90 minutes.

5. Eat More Protein for Breakfast

If you're cutting back on the above, then what *should* you eat for breakfast? The answer is more *protein and vegetables*. Don't worry about the fat that comes along with it. The breakfast that I recommend starts with eggs.

My preference for breakfast is either two or three eggs boiled, fried, scrambled, or poached—without toast. I will almost always add a vegetable—most often cauliflower—to my breakfast and put butter on the vegetable.

Add bacon freely to your breakfast. As long as you have no starchy carbs or sweets, the bacon will have only a miniscule impact on your blood sugar and weight.

Now when should you eat an egg-white omelet and when should you eat a whole-egg omelet? I'll eat an egg-white omelet if I'm going to do a strength workout because an egg-white omelet usually has the whites of six or seven eggs—that means 42 to 49 grams of protein, whereas a whole-egg omelet usually consists of three complete eggs, and has only 21 grams of protein. More protein will help you improve the ratio of muscle to fat whether you are a man or woman.

When I say that fat will not significantly add to your blood sugar or weight, that's true as long as you don't eat starchy or sweet carbs with the meal. Here's more specific timing. *Based on my blood sugar testing, I've learned that in order to keep your blood low after eating fat,* **you should not eat starchy or sweet carbs one hour before a meal** *with fat in it,* *during a meal with fat in it, or* **three hours after the meal** *with fat in it.*

6. Eat Vegetables for Breakfast

Who eats vegetables for breakfast? The truth is not many Americans do unless they are making a veggie omelet—which by the way is a great weight-loss breakfast. But by not eating a vegetable for breakfast, we're missing out on a great health addition for our first meal of the day.

I stopped eating toast and started eating tomato slices for breakfast years ago. Then I moved into different vegetables. Now I often have a healthy portion of either asparagus, broccoli, or cauliflower, each with melted butter. Once I started that habit, I started losing weight quickly even though that wasn't necessarily my goal. My goal was better blood glucose control, but as you now know, if you control your glucose, you control your weight.

Like the fat in bacon and eggs, the butter fat will have little impact on your blood sugar. Switching away from starchy carbs for breakfast and to protein and vegetables with or without butter is one of the easiest and most effective ways to reduce blood sugar and lose weight. I choose to use butter with my vegetables because vegetables taste so much better with butter. My daily consumption of vegetables has gone up and my blood glucose and weight have gone down.

In Summary, Follow This Pattern for Breakfast

- Dilute your juices.

- Eliminate *starchy carbohydrates* such as bread, muffins, cereal, and potatoes.

- Do not eat sweet rolls, donuts, or any other *sweet carbohydrates* for breakfast.

- Eat more *protein* and *fat*.

- Start adding a *vegetable or vegetables* to your breakfast.

If you start that breakfast eating pattern you *will* start losing weight because the glucose from those foods will go very slowly into your bloodstream and you'll have three or more hours to burn that glucose before it's stored around your body in all the places you don't want it stored: mostly stomach for men, and legs and hips for women.

That slow entry into your bloodstream also results in a much more diminished sense of hunger at lunch than you would have if you had eaten cereal, bagels, or any other starchy carbs. You will be less likely to eat a big lunch.

But breakfast is just one part of the eating equation. The other three parts are lunch, dinner, and snacks. Next let's look at lunch.

Lunch

1. Minimize Starchy Carbs for Lunch

Once again, do everything you can to minimize starchy carbs.

At lunch time, starchy carbs often enter your eating patterns in the form of bread on sandwiches, buns on burgers or hot dogs, rolls, bagels, French fries, potato chips, taco shells, tortilla chips, rice, and pasta.

A note on bread: White bread and multigrain bread all have a similar high impact on blood sugar and weight gain. Whole-grain or whole wheat are slightly better for you and have slightly less impact on blood sugar than multigrain or white bread. If you can't shake the bread habit, then eat only small portions and only whole wheat bread.

2. Eliminate Dessert from Lunch

Most desserts are combinations of sweet and starchy carbs such as cakes and pies or combinations of sweet and fatty carbs such as ice cream. Remember those combinations are blood-sugar-raising, weight-gaining bombshells. Do not eat dessert for lunch.

3. Eat Plenty of Protein, Fat, and Veggie Carbs for Lunch

Don't worry about holding back on protein, fat, or veggie carbs for lunch. Remember a salad consists mostly of veggie carbs and you can put dressing on the salad with impunity as long as you don't eat any starchy carbs (including croutons) or have any sweets just before lunch, during lunch, or for three hours after lunch.

Most people already *know* how good vegetables are for you, but I'll repeat again what most people *don't know* that's even better. Veggie carbs— especially with butter are so slow to enter your bloodstream as glucose, you are likely to burn that glucose before it's ever stored as body fat.

Eating protein, fat (but not potato chips), and vegetables (but not French fries) for lunch will help you eliminate snacking in the afternoon and leave you less hungry by dinnertime. Enjoy as much as you want from those three groups.

4. Fruit is Okay for Lunch

If you follow my suggestions above but do have fruit with your lunch, it will be only a slight diminishing of weight-loss of the protein, fat, and vegetables. If you do eat fruit, do not eat too much. The best fruits for any meal are blueberries, blackberries, raspberries, or cantaloupe.

But if fruit is your biggest weight contributor for lunch you are going to do fine and continue to lose weight.

If you followed the Glucose Control Eating© eating pattern for breakfast, you won't be as hungry at lunchtime and by following the pattern I'm now describing for lunch, you won't be as hungry at dinnertime. That also means you'll be less likely to snack after these meals.

I do realize that it's not always a sense of hunger that dictates whether we snack or not. Often, we snack just for something to do. I talk more about this later.

In Summary, Follow these Glucose Control Eating© Steps for Lunch.

- Minimize *starchy* carbs at lunch.

- Eliminate sweet carbs (any sugars and desserts) at lunch.

- Eat *protein, fat,* and *veggie carbs* at lunch.

- A limited amount of fruit is okay.

Dinner

Dinner is the meal that is the biggest contributor to weight gain in America and it's the meal that is *least* likely to have its calories burned by post-meal activity, plus it's the meal most likely to have dessert associated with it.

In chapter 11, on modest increases in your activity, I talk about the importance of getting at least 15 minutes of some activity between dinner and going to bed. Whether it's walking, shopping, gardening, or just moving around the house more, that activity between dinner and bedtime will have a disproportionally high weight-loss benefit.

More activity after dinner is, of course, better but even a small amount will make a difference as you will learn later.

I don't recommend eating fatty foods as freely for dinner as I do for breakfast or lunch because fat takes as long as three to four hours to slowly get into your bloodstream. That is good for breakfast and lunch, because the fat goes in so slowly that you can burn it in your daily activity. But if you eat dinner too late, the glucose from the fatty foods will be going into your body while you are sleeping and that, of course, is not good. You burn so little glucose while you sleep that most of this glucose will not be used. It *will* be stored as fat.

I was eating dinner with a friend recently and he said, "Look at you. You don't even have to think about what you eat for dinner." My answer was short and quick. "That's not correct. I've been thinking about what I eat for 30 years." It's true. I rarely sit down for dinner and just "dig in." At meals I'm always thinking about minimizing starchy carbs, sweet carbs (dessert), and at a late dinner I also think about moderating fat. The key word here is *moderating* fat, not eliminating it.

We all desire some starchy carbs at times, and we are all going to have desserts periodically. But the important issue –you are now aware of— is the huge impact that both sweet carbs and starchy carbs will have on your blood glucose and on weight gain.

Think of it this way. If the price of gasoline were to go up by two dollars a gallon tomorrow, we probably would not just flat-out stop driving, but we would be much more cautious about how much we would drive. Before we get in our cars, we would likely think about the impact on our pocketbooks.

Think about starchy carbs and sweet carbs like that. We are all going to eat them from time to time, but before you do, think about the impact on your blood glucose and weight. Just keep minimizing those blood glucose elevators until their minimization ultimately becomes your habit.

If we're having a special dinner with warm, aromatic rolls being passed around the dinner table, I'm going to have one—with butter, of course, even though I know that's not good for blood glucose or weight.

If we're having company for dinner and a dessert is served, I will, sometimes, have a small portion. These small enjoyments are an important part of life. I haven't given them up completely and you don't have to either. But remember— make them special, make them small, make them infrequent—*not part of your regular dinner routine.*

What should you eat for dinner? The good thing about breaking down foods into the six groups instead of just three is that you now know which *food groups* you can *maximize* and which *food groups* you should *minimize*. With that knowledge, lowering your blood glucose, losing weight, and keeping it off will be much easier.

1. Minimize *starchy* carbs for dinner just like you do for all other meals

Here is where you must be careful of the two veggie carbs that act like starchy carbs—corn and potatoes. You do not have to eliminate them, just minimize them.

Minimize or eliminate breads, rolls, and rice, and pasta. In all these foods the brown versions are just slightly better than white versions. But work hard at eliminating all starchy carbs except for special meals.

2. Some Fruit Is Okay

In terms of weight gain, you now know that fruit is somewhere in between the good groups—protein, fat, and vegetables—and the bad groups—sweet and starchy carbs. So be cautious and try to stick with berries and cantaloupe.

Go ahead and have fruit with or after dinner if you choose, but don't overindulge and don't put the fruit on ice cream more than a couple of times a year.

3. Freely Eat Protein and Veggie Carbs at Dinner As Well As Fat under Specific Conditions

Fish, poultry, meat, and veggie carbohydrates should be the core of your dinner. The skin is okay on poultry and fat is okay on meat. But dinner is when you should minimize butter on vegetables, fish, or any seafood. If you are going to have some fat for dinner you need to avoid starchy and sweet carbs in that meal and eat your dinner at least three hours before going to bed.

At home I have typical dinners of grilled, blackened, or baked Alaskan salmon, cod, or halibut. Crab and shrimp are also two of my favorites. These seafoods, plus pollock and lobster, have an almost negligible impact on blood sugar and weight.

A few times a month we'll have chicken or meat instead of fish. Both chicken—including the skin but not breading—and red meat are good for keeping blood sugar low and weight down if you do not have starchy carbs in the same meal or sweet carbs for dessert.

My veggie carbs are typically broccoli, cauliflower, asparagus, green beans, and a variety of mixed salads with lettuce, vegetables, nuts, and fruit topped with blue cheese dressing. All good.

Timing at Dinner

A significant concern about having fat for dinner is how slow the fat makes its way into your bloodstream compared to the other food groups.

- **Sweet carbs** get into your bloodstream within three to ten minutes and most often get stored as body fat before you can burn the glucose they create.

- **Starchy carbs** get into your bloodstream in 5 to 30 minutes. Unless you're exercising or very active after eating, they will also be stored as body fat.

- **Protein and Veggie carbs** create much less glucose and go in much slower—20 to 90 minutes. If you have 15 to 30 minutes of casual activity such as walking, gardening, or shopping after dinner, you'll have sufficient time to burn the glucose they create before it's stored.

- **Fat** is the slowest of all foods to enter your bloodstream. It takes from two to five hours to break down and enter the bloodstream as glucose. That's good if you eat fat for breakfast, lunch, or an early dinner because you'll have plenty of time to burn the glucose it creates before it ever has a chance to be stored as body fat. But that is bad if you eat a late dinner and go to sleep within an hour or two after eating. The fat will continue going into your bloodstream as glucose while you're sleeping and your blood sugar will continue rising for the first few hours you're sleeping. The glucose the fat creates will *not get* burned as it will after breakfast, lunch, or an early dinner, but some *will* get stored as body fat.

Remember if you eat an *early* dinner (three or more hours before you go to bed), you can eat a small amount of meat with fat or fish with butter. You can also put a small amount of butter on vegetables. An early dinner is much better than a late dinner for lowering your weight. If you do eat a late dinner, you should minimize fat.

4. Reduce Portion Sizes for Dinner

Portion size for dinner is more important than portion size for breakfast and lunch. It's the meal you're least likely to burn and most likely to store as fat simply because you usually will not have as much activity after dinner as you have after breakfast or lunch.

At first, you will find it hard to think about dinner as a small meal. As a child and a teenager at home I remember my dad would finish a big dinner, typically of fried chicken, roast beef, or meat loaf with mashed potatoes and gravy, often with corn and biscuits and then lean back in his chair and declare with great satisfaction, "I feel like a million bucks." It was his way of saying he was full and, as a child of the depression, being full was good to Dad.

You may have grown up with the same messages I heard frequently. "Take all you want but eat all you take." "Clean your plate." "Eat your potatoes." The intent was all positive but when you heard it over and over you couldn't help but think eating a lot is good and not eating very much is bad.

If you can adopt a mindset that being full after dinner is not necessarily good and act on that, you will be well on your way to losing weight.

I know this is not easy but if you can start making smaller dinners your pattern, it will eventually become your habit. You will slip and backslide a little as you start making dinner a smaller meal. Don't say, "I failed and can't do this." Promise yourself you'll do better tomorrow.

Here's a comment I got from a reader of my previous book about Type 2 diabetes. I love the fact that he admits to occasional bad days.

> I'm a two-year Type II diabetic and have been following your diet and lifestyle recommendations (with occasional "bad" days) since I was first diagnosed. Now, for the first time in 30 years all my bloodwork was in the normal range. A1C was 5.3, liver enzymes low normal, total cholesterol down, good cholesterol up, my weight is down 40 pounds since February. I was supposed to start taking Metformin [a blood-glucose-lowering medication] but due to some surgeries that prescription was postponed. At my recent annual physical,

my doctor said don't bother with that medication, your A1C of 5.3 is in the normal, nondiabetic range. You're no longer a borderline diabetic.

Chuck Culver
Anchorage, Alaska

Remember, you do not have to be perfect. You just have to be good.

Two suggestions for starting the habit of "dinner as a smaller meal"

1. Make a promise to yourself to eat your dinner for one month from a dessert plate. This will constantly remind you of your goal to make dinner a smaller meal. If you can do that for one month, you'll find yourself eating less and feeling better right away. When you feel you know what a smaller dinner is and when you think you can continue eating smaller even if your plate is bigger, go back to a normal dinner plate. You'll find a feeling of pride as your dinner plate actually has spaces among your helpings of food.

2. Start making a checkmark for each day you're successful in making dinner a small meal. Maybe the first week you'll be successful for only three dinners out of seven. The next week shoot for four or five days of success with your new pattern. Keep on doing that until you've succeeded all seven days in a week. Then shoot for a second consecutive week of that pattern. Once you get to four consecutive weeks, *you will have lost a lot of weight and be close to making small dinners your habit.*

You Can Do It

Eating the foods I recommend in smaller portion sizes will not only help you start losing weight and gaining control of your blood sugar right away, but more importantly, it can become a healthy eating habit that will help keep you lean and trim for the rest of your life.

I make a special point throughout these chapters of saying "typical" dinners and not "every" dinner because we all want special dinners on occasion. That's simply an important part of life. Don't give those times up. Enjoy them but even on those special times don't go overboard on starchy carbohydrates or desserts.

How about Snacking

There is a danger, however, in smaller dinner portions. The temptation to snack after dinner and before you go to bed will be even greater. How can you deal with that temptation?

After-Dinner Snacks

I've talked about breakfast, lunch, and dinner. Of those three meals, dinner is the meal most likely to contribute to weight gain. But right up there with dinner as a big contributor to weight gain is what's eaten after dinner—evening snacks.

Like dinner, an evening snack is a habit that is less likely to be followed by activity. When you're snacking after dinner you may be contributing mightily to blood glucose increases and weight gain. After years and years of testing my blood sugar after dinner while sometimes snacking and sometimes not, here are my seven conclusions.

1. After-dinner snacks are bigger contributors to weight gain and blood sugar increases than are post-breakfast and post-lunch snacks. This may be an obvious conclusion simply because we're all more likely to burn some glucose from snacks we eat at 10 a.m. or 3 p.m. than snacks we eat at 8 or 9 p.m. Those late-evening snacks are much more likely to be stored as fat than burned.

   I've never been in the habit of eating a midmorning or midafternoon snack and I don't recommend it, but they are not as impactful on weight and blood glucose as a post-dinner snack.

2. If you are going to snack after dinner, stay away from ice cream or potato chips. They will not only raise your blood glucose (and weight) because of the sweet and starchy carbs, but also, because of their fat content. They will both continue to increase your blood glucose for four or more hours after you eat them. By that time, you're likely going to be asleep and subject to the worst-case scenario of increasing blood sugar while you're burning very few calories and therefore subjecting yourself to increasing weight gain during the night.

3. If you feel you must snack, the best by far is a veggie selection or some protein. My favorite veggie snacks are broccoli, cauliflower, carrots and radishes with blue cheese dressing. A moderate amount of dressing is okay as long as you don't have any starchy carbs such as crackers with it. For protein snacks, I like smoked salmon, shrimp, or reindeer sausage.

4. A good way to improve your snacks is, "Don't buy the bad stuff." If you do buy ice cream, potato chips, candy, and similar snacks—whether you keep them visible or try to hide them from yourself—*you will eat them.* It's easier to resist them at the grocery store than to resist them in your home.

5. My next suggestion is to ask yourself when you're most likely to eat sweet or starchy snacks. I'm guessing it's when you're watching TV or in front of your computer. Before you sit down, ask yourself what else you could snack on besides sweets. Right now, as I'm writing this, I'm snacking on walnuts I roasted yesterday for a salad yesterday.

6. Even with healthier snacks do not eat them by the handful. Eat them one at a time and take a little time in between. I've learned over the years to eat snacks less frequently and more slowly and savor each bite a little more. By doing that you will automatically be eating a little less. It's a good pattern to get into and soon you'll find it has become a habit.

7. An excellent way to take temptation out of snacking after dinner is to start with what I refer to as a V-8 cocktail. It's very simply V-8 juice and sparking mineral water like Perrier or Pellegrino or Safeway's brand, Signature. In a full-size glass, mix the liquids to your taste. I like about 50% V-8. At 50% V-8 you're getting only 22 calories. I usually drink two glasses a day of that V-8 cocktail and if you wish you can add Bloody Mary-like spices to the mixture. It's healthy—according to the label that amount would be equivalent to two servings of vegetables. You will feel full and have less desire to snack on anything else.

8. V-8 also has a low-sodium version as well as a spicy version. V-8 juice is a good friend of weight loss.

The best plan of all is *not to snack after dinner.* If you can accomplish that you will have taken one of the biggest weight-loss steps possible.

In Summary, Follow These Glucose Control Eating© Patterns for Dinner.

- Eat Dinner as Early as You Reasonably Can.

- Minimize Starchy Carbs Just Like You Do for Other Meals.

- Eliminate Sweet Carbs (Desserts) after Dinner.

- Some fruits are okay but moderate them.

- Freely eat protein and veggie carbs at dinner.

- Moderate fat with early dinners and minimize or eliminate fat with late dinners.

- Reduce portion sizes for dinner.

- Minimize or eliminate after-dinner snacks.

Chapter 8

Tips on Losing Weight When Eating Out

Why I Haven't Included "Breakfast Out" in This Section

Breakfast choices are typically much narrower than lunch and dinner choices. Any discussion about *eating breakfasts out* would be much the same as eating breakfast at home and therefore repetitive.

Lunch Out

Good Lunch Choices at National-Franchise Sit-Down Restaurants

As you begin lowering blood glucose and losing weight by cutting back on sweets, and starchy carbs, and adding protein, vegetables, and fat, here are some thoughts on restaurant options.

Here's my suggestion for a healthier lunch technique if I'm eating in franchise restaurants like Chili's, TGIF, Appleby's, Red Robin and so forth. I'll order a hamburger, a fish sandwich (not breaded), a chicken sandwich, or a turkey sandwich all *without the top bun.* I'll always ask if they have an alternative to French fries. If they don't, then I'll do without anything but the burger because once French fries make it to your plate, they will also make it to your mouth. Most of the time, however, you will be able to get a vegetable alternative. It's an opportunity to have another helping of some vegetable.

When you get your food, use your knife and fork to eat the meat, chicken, turkey, or fish and the onions, tomatoes, and lettuce in the sandwich, then leave the bottom half of the sandwich on your plate. By leaving both halves of the bun behind, you've contributed greatly to lowering blood glucose and losing weight. Even if you take a bite or two of the bun or bread, you are still doing fine.

This, of course, also holds true for lunch at any other restaurant that serves lunch. I just used national-franchise restaurants as an example because of their standardized menus.

Fast-Food Restaurants

Like most people I find myself at fast food restaurants occasionally. For me that's one or two times a month. Eating too often at fast food restaurants can be a problem—but not necessarily. Here are my recommendations for ways to eat fast foods that will keep your blood glucose and weight down.

Arby's

Arby's has a roast beef sandwich that I really like. Here's my pattern for eating it. I always ask for one of their plastic forks. Then I sit down, take the top half of the bun off and just eat the roast beef with Arby's horsey sauce and when I'm done I throw both halves of the bun away. That has very little impact on my blood sugar or insulin demand and I'm always amazed at how they can make roast beef so tender and juicy.

Carl's Jr

Carl's Jr. will do all their burger choices in a low-carb format. That's one of my favorite fast-food burgers. It's simply any of their burgers wrapped in lettuce instead of a bun. That diminishes dramatically the impact it has on blood sugar glucose and weight. It's a little too big so I don't always eat it all and have quit trying to eat it in my car as takeout. The lettuce wrap is not as neat as a bun and it can be messy. I usually sit down in the restaurant and eat it there. You get a lot of meat and vegetables and you won't be hungry again until dinner.

Subway
Subway offers a lot of choices. Now that you know about veggie carbs and protein you can use that information in your selections. My pattern is to order the 6-inch instead of the 12-inch sandwich then just eat one half or less of the bun. You know by now, the less of the bun you eat the better for your weight loss.

Mexican Restaurants
Most Mexican foods as prepared in Mexican restaurants in America have a lot of fat, starchy carbs, and some protein as primary ingredients, a generally bad combination for anyone who wants to lose weight.

I usually eat fajitas or a queen tostada which have the protein and vegetables separated and easily eaten without having to eat the starchy-carb wrappings—you should do that. I will also eat tacos and try to leave as much of the shell as I can on the plate. Also, cut way back or eliminate the refried beans and rice as they are very starchy and will have a big impact on your blood glucose and weight.

Dinner Out

Portion Size—the Biggest Problem in
Most American Restaurants
About 20 years ago I had flown down from Alaska to visit my mom in southern California. Instead of flying home after the visit, I decided to do something a little different and take a train, the Sunset Limited, from Los Angeles to Seattle and then fly home to Alaska from Seattle. As the train rolled north through the hills of the San Joaquin Valley, I sat down at a nicely set table in the dining car for lunch and was joined by a Dutch couple. They had been touring America by auto and were now taking the train to Seattle to catch a flight home to Holland.

They were very pleasant, congenial, and open people. Unfortunately, I've forgotten their names, so I'll just call them Mr. and Mrs. Holland. I asked them the obvious question, "What's your impression of America?" With no hesitation, Mrs. Holland blurted out, "Big." I said, "Big? Well, yes America is a big country." She said, "No, it's not just the country—it's everything. Everything's big." I knew they had talked between themselves about this because Mr. Holland continued her thought. "The mountains are big. The roads are big. The cars are big. The people are big, and the food in the restaurants is big."

Well, I'd never heard anyone call restaurant food "big," but they continued laughing and describing a litany of the large portions of food that they had been served at the last half dozen restaurants they had patronized along their journey.

In the years since that conversation, I've become more sensitive to portion sizes in restaurants. The Dutch couple was correct. The portions in American restaurants are very big.

If you eat in restaurants a lot, cutting back on the portion sizes, eating fewer starchy carbs, and ordering dessert only for special occasions are essential patterns you need to start and turn into habits if you want lose weight.

Tips for Reducing Portion Size

By now you know the general guidelines for what to eat. So I'm going to focus on portion size, which I believe is a big problem for most of us when we eat dinner out.

Here are three effective ways to reduce portion size in restaurants:

1. Share the entrée with your dinner partner. This idea is becoming more common especially with restaurant dinner customers in their 50s and older, but it's a good idea for anyone of any age who wants to lose weight. Some restaurants will, however, charge a second-plate fee but many do not.

2. Make an appetizer (or maybe three appetizers for two of you) your dinner following the Glucose Control Eating© guidelines. If you try this for a few months as a pattern and are able to let it evolve into a habit, you will have achieved a great health victory and be on your way to significant weight loss, and dramatically improved health. Make no mistake about this. It is hard. This is a time you'll need to motivate yourself to get the positive results you will experience.

3. If you order a full meal, as you place your order, ask the server to put half the meal in a to-go container before he or she brings it out to you. You'll find it so much easier to only eat half of the overly generous plateful of food if you don't see the other half until you look in the refrigerator the next day.

A Final Thought on a Seafood Restaurant and Butter

Seafood restaurants provide the best opportunity to illustrate a delicious way to enjoy good size servings of protein, vegetables, and fat with insignificant increases in blood sugar and weight.

One of my favorite chain restaurants is Red Lobster, a seafood restaurant that I eat at when I'm in California or Arizona. Over the years I've eaten there I've confirmed—by consistent blood sugar testing before and after meals there—that I can eat all the lobster, prawns, scallops, salmon, halibut, and vegetables that I want with all the melted butter, with almost negligible impact on my blood glucose and weight.

However, once again, I must stress that all that changes if I eat starchy carbs with the meal or follow the meal with sweet carbs. But if you stay away from those two groups it's a wonderful way to enjoy a delicious, healthy, weight-loss meal.

Chapter 9

The Glucose Control
Eating Grid©

Eating Lifestyle Changes—Comparing Degrees of
Difficulty to Degrees of Benefit

You'll see in this chapter that some of the Glucose Control Eating© changes are very easy, some are slightly harder. You'll also find that the degrees of benefit vary. Some changes in your diet will make a small difference in your blood glucose, weight, and health in the short run but will still be significant in the long run. Other changes will have a bigger benefit right away and will be even more significant over the months and years. And some changes will have a dramatic impact on your weight very quickly and be life-changing over the years.

You'll stumble or falter a bit along the way, but the results will be worth it. Remember, each of these changes is part of the whole package of eating changes that together will give you a healthier life. You don't have to embrace and adopt them all but the more of them you do adopt, the healthier and leaner you'll be. Nor do you have to be perfect in your eating lifestyle—only good.

Explaining the Glucose Control Grid©
I struggled for a long time on how to present these actions by ease or difficulty of the action and significance of the benefit. Should I assign a number, sort of like degree of difficulty in diving or gymnastics? That didn't work, because it implied a degree of specificity that was not

defensible. The same applied with the degree of benefit. How do you assign a valid numeric value to the different changes I've recommended? Finally, I came up with the idea of a glucose control weight-loss grid. Along the horizontal axis (X axis) is the degree of difficulty (to the right is harder) and along the vertical axis (Y axis) is the degree of benefit (up is more weight loss benefit).

I have 18 weight-loss actions listed below. Think about each of those actions and then consider where they are placed in the weight-loss grid. Then decide which of those actions you want to start with. The more actions you take, the faster your weight loss will be.

If you're really serious about losing weight fast, take note of the eating actions I put **in bold type**. If you can adopt those actions, your body fat will seem to just melt away.

When you reach your desired weight, don't go back to your old way of eating—instead, just slide back to some of the nonbolded actions.

As you look at the Glucose Control Grid©, you'll see that the single action in the lower left quadrant of the grid is easy and has moderate weight-loss benefit. Those actions in the upper left quadrant are still easy but have more benefit and those actions in the upper right quadrant are more difficult but also have significant benefit.

In the lower left quadrant is only one action, but it's very easy and yet has pretty good benefit. In the upper left quadrant are six actions. All fairly easy but with good weight-loss results. The upper right quadrant has eleven actions, all big contributors to weight loss. These actions are somewhat harder but will have great short- and long-term benefits. These are the changes that you will have to work at, but if you're successful at achieving them, they can be life-changing.

Finally, in the lower right-hand quadrant would be changes that are hard but would have little or no benefit. I haven't even discussed anything that conceivably might fit in that quadrant (difficult but of no benefit) and would have no reason to do so.

In all quadrants, the higher the number is placed, the greater the benefit and the farther right the number is placed, the more difficult.

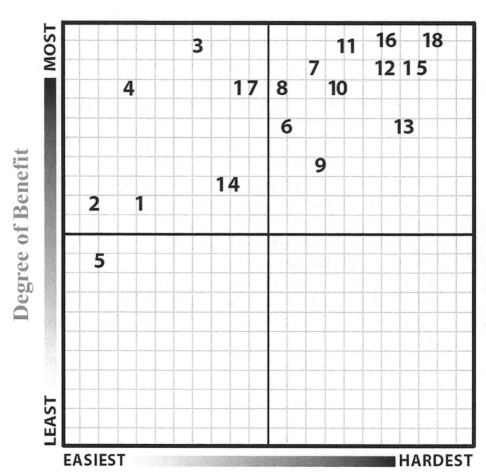

Breakfast

1. Reduce starchy carbs in your breakfast.

2. Eat egg-white omelets if you have any starchy carbs at all.

3. **Eliminate starchy carbs from your breakfast—no cereal, no toast or muffins, no potatoes.**

4. **Add more protein and vegetables to your breakfast—whole eggs and butter are okay if you eat no sweet or starchy carbs.**

5. **Dilute your breakfast juices.**

Lunch

6. Reduce starchy carbs in your lunches and eat more protein and vegetables.

7. **Eliminate starchy carbs at lunch and eat only protein, fat, vegetables, and maybe a small amount of fruit for lunch—butter and salad dressing are okay.**

8. Eliminate desserts at lunch.

Dinner

9. **Eat dinner earlier.**

10. Eat more protein and vegetables and fewer starchy carbs for dinner.

11. **Eat only protein, vegetables, and a small portion of fruit for dinner** *butter and salad dressings are okay if you eat at least three hours before going to sleep.*

12. **Reduce portion size for dinner at home and in restaurants.**

13. Share an entree with your dinner partner at restaurants.

14. Order an appetizer—or maybe two—in place of dinner at restaurants.

15. Ask for half of your meal to be put in a to-go box before you get it.

After-Dinner Snacks

16. **Eliminate eating desserts as a regular habit—special occasions are okay.**

17. Improve and/or reduce your after-dinner snacks.

18. **Eliminate your after-dinner snacks.**

Conclusion

Review the changes listed and then review the location of each change on the Glucose Control Weight Loss graph. After you've considered the benefit and the ease or difficulty of those changes, decide which you want to include in your Glucose Control Eating©. The more actions you take, the faster your weight loss will be.

Once you start the eating pattern of Glucose Control Eating©, you will start lowering your blood glucose and losing weight right away. When you continue that eating pattern you will continue losing weight. If you are losing too much weight just back off one or two of your actions.

Losing weight and becoming healthier is about changing lifestyles. It's about setting new patterns of eating and then making those patterns habits.

At first, you'll have to think about it every day. It will be easier now that you know which foods to eat and which to avoid. But when you follow these patterns for a few weeks, the patterns will become habits and you won't even have to think about it.

When you wake up in the morning, you don't look at a note that says, "Brush your teeth and wash your face." You don't need to think about getting a cup of coffee, getting the newspaper from your porch or opening the news up on your tablet, or having your normal breakfast. You just do it. And you certainly don't need a note that says, "Say good morning," to your husband, wife, or partner. You've established certain patterns and they've just become habits.

Make Glucose Control Eating© your habit and you will keep your weight off for the rest of your life.

Chapter 10

Obesity, Diabetes, and Why You Need Glucose Control Eating© *Now*

If you are *significantly* overweight or obese now, you know the physical and emotional challenges you face every day.

I don't presume to know those challenges as well as you do so I'm not going to dwell on them here. But in this chapter, I do talk about problems you may face as you get older if you don't lose weight now.

If you are just *moderately* overweight, you probably feel less agile, less energetic and a more tired during the day than you did before you gained the weight. You may also be less confident about your appearance.

If you're just *slightly* overweight, you may not notice or feel any different than before you gained the weight but you're probably aware and a little concerned about your weight creepage.

If you fit into one of those three categories of overweight, it may be some small comfort to know that you are not alone. Currently, an estimated 42% of American adults are obese. Another 33% are considered moderately or slightly overweight leaving about 23% for the normal or healthy weight category and about 2% in the underweight group.

While these numbers are hard to quantify for obvious reasons, all the estimates I have seen from various health groups seem to reflect similar numbers.

Whether you are slightly, moderately, or significantly overweight, you're more knowledgeable than I am about the current challenges you face but you may not know about what you could face in the future.

Knowing that the vast majority of Americans have the same problem as you doesn't mitigate the upcoming health problems you may face in the near or long-term future. In this chapter, I'll alert you to the epidemic of Type 2 diabetes in the United States and its avoidance or reversal.

———

Type 2 diabetes and the complications that often accompany it are serious problems. But Type 2 diabetes is avoidable—or if you already have it—it is reversible.

Importantly, Glucose Control Eating© is not only a successful weight-loss diet, but it is also the eating lifestyle needed to avoid or reverse Type 2 diabetes.

In fact, the Glucose Control Eating© was developed as a Type 2 diabetes reversal diet. It worked. Throughout Alaska, borderline diabetics, pre-diabetics, and full-blown Type 2 diabetics raved about the success they experienced with Glucose Control Eating©. (When I first developed this eating lifestyle, it was called, *The Diabetes Lifeline Diet*). While they were proud of their blood glucose reduction and their Type 2 diabetes reversal, they were effusive in their comments about weight loss.

To help motivate you in your weight-loss journey, I'll share this article from *The Week* magazine that very concisely lists the problems faced by obese adults.

In an article titled "The Obesity Epidemic", *The Week* magazine on October 19, 2019, headlined, "A public health emergency is shortening our lives and supersizing our health-care costs."

As obesity surged over the past three decades, US diabetes rates tripled, and now more than 100 million adults have diabetes or pre-diabetes. Research suggests that obese people are between 1.5 and 2 times more likely to die of heart disease. Other illnesses linked to obesity include high blood pressure, arthritis, Alzheimer's disease, gallbladder disease, sleep apnea, sexual dysfunction, and at least 13 types of cancer. The American Cancer Society believes excess weight is linked to about 7 percent of cancer deaths, and obesity will soon overtake smoking as the top preventable cause of cancer.

All these maladies have some association with being overweight, but the one most directly associated with being overweight is Type 2 diabetes. Being overweight as you get older dramatically increases the likelihood of your getting Type 2 diabetes.

Weight Gain and the Type 2 Diabetic Epidemic

It's no coincidence that about two-thirds of Americans are overweight and about one-third of American adults have Type 2 diabetes and another third are borderline diabetic. If bad eating habits and being overweight are the most common causes of Type 2 diabetes, why are there almost twice as many overweight people as Type 2 diabetics? The answer is simple. People first gain weight then begin having indicators of Type 2 diabetes—referred to as pre-diabetics or borderline diabetics.

Many argue that the rate of increase of Type 2 diabetes puts it in the category of an epidemic, although unlike other more infamous epidemics such as the bubonic plague, influenza, cholera, and smallpox, it doesn't pose the likelihood of immediate death. It does, however, pose the likelihood of a significantly shortened and unhealthy life.

Not only will unchecked Type 2 diabetes significantly shorten life span, but the precursors to diabetes and the additional weight associated with it may have already started the life-shortening process.

How important is weight in this epidemic? First, not all Type 2 diabetics are overweight and not all overweight people have Type 2 diabetes. Type 2 diabetes may in some cases be hereditary and may in some cases be culturally influenced, *but without question the most common characteristic associated with Type 2 diabetics is being overweight.*

Consequently, losing weight is the best action you can take to avoid Type 2 diabetes. Almost all Type 2 diabetics would like to lose weight. But that is much easier hoped for than done.

To cure or reverse Type 2 diabetes, or to avoid getting Type 2 diabetes in the first place, you need an understanding of the disease, a desire to be healthy, a positive attitude, and knowledge of what foods you should be eating.

The understanding of what foods you should be eating is precisely what you have learned in this book. That understanding can be life-changing for you.

To give you a little more motivation to put that knowledge into practice and make those healthy changes in your eating habits, this next section will highlight some problems you may face if you don't keep your blood glucose and weight under control.

If you're an overweight person, it's important for you to know something about diabetes in general and to know the difference between Type 1 and Type 2 diabetes.

Type 1 and Type 2 diabetes are two different versions of the same disease. Type 1—which is what I have had for 58 years—is not reversible, but it is manageable. Type 2 is reversible with the Glucose Control Diet©.

The Difference Between Type 1 and Type 2 Diabetes

Here's a story I use periodically in my speeches. By the time you finish this book anyone who is a Type 2 diabetic will fully understand and appreciate the truth of this short parable.

A Type 1 diabetic and a Type 2 diabetic are marooned on a desert island. Neither has any insulin; however, they do have a way to make fires and the island does have catchable fish, edible plants, and drinkable water.

Despite access to the nourishment needed to survive, but with no insulin, the Type 1 diabetic would be dead in a month. In that same length of time, the Type 2 diabetic would be cured.

Now, I don't expect anyone to just eat plants and fish and drink water, but you don't have to. You now have the tools to reverse or avoid ever getting Type 2 diabetes.

I'll talk briefly about Type 1 diabetes just to give you an understanding of the difference between the two types of diabetes.

AUTHOR'S NOTE:
I use the word "cure" in the parable because having normal blood sugars is the very definition of a nondiabetic. Some may argue that "cure" is the wrong word because even if blood sugars are normalized the former diabetic may be more susceptible to becoming a Type 2 diabetic again if old habits return. But whether it is called "cured" or "reversed," the likelihood of diabetic complications is dramatically diminished and a longer, healthier life is the result.

Type 1 diabetes

Type 1 diabetes is most often diagnosed between birth and about age 25. It is not related to eating or exercise habits.

The pancreas just stops producing insulin, which is a hormone that allows the glucose created by the food that has been eaten to get from the bloodstream to the cells for energy. Without insulin, the glucose cannot get out of the bloodstream into the cells to provide energy for immediate use or for storage for future use.

Within the constraints of today's technology, Type 1 is not curable, but it is very manageable. And good management allows for a healthy, productive, and long life. As a long-term Type 1 diabetic, I owe my healthy life to what I've learned about eating right and to the development of the tools and technology that allow me to measure and control the glucose in my bloodstream.

Type 2 Diabetes

Now let's focus on Type 2 diabetes. After giving presentations to thousands of Type 2 diabetics, I have come to consider Type 2 as more serious and resulting in a shorter life span from the onset than Type 1 does.

When people get Type 1 diabetes, they are usually young and healthy, and the onset is typically not related to bad eating habits or a sedentary life. Because they are young and healthy, they have more time to understand the disease and get it under control.

But when people get Type 2, they are older and often have years or decades of not-so-good eating habits and/or a sedentary life. Their organs and circulatory systems are not as healthy as those of the younger Type 1 diabetics and therefore, they have less time before the diabetes complications start damaging their bodies. That's why it is urgent for Type 2s to act promptly to get their blood glucose under control.

The good news about Type 2, however, is that it can be reversed.

If you learn to control your blood glucose, you will control your weight… and you will avoid or reverse Type 2 diabetes.

Type 2 is typically—but not always—diagnosed at an older age, most commonly 40s through 70s or even 80s. It is usually—but not always—associated with eating the wrong foods combined with a relatively inactive lifestyle.

Because of less-than-healthy eating habits, the quantity of glucose (sugar) in the bloodstream is higher and requires the pancreas to work harder to produce more insulin to get the blood sugar back to normal levels. The pancreas is in effect "overworked" and eventually can't produce enough insulin to get all the excess glucose out of the bloodstream into the cells.

The result is higher than normal blood sugars (glucose). And if you don't correct that and bring your blood glucose down to normal levels soon, you'll have to deal with all the serious complications brought on by high blood glucose over time.

Over and over I hear the same quiet and melancholy reflections from middle-aged and older Type 2 diabetics who may be suffering from circulatory problems, kidney failure, serious vision problems, foot sores, foot ulcers, and potential amputations, "I should have taken my high blood sugars more seriously." Or "I wish I had been more conscientious about my blood glucose years ago." It's sad to hear those comments but they are very understandable.

Why Are High Blood Sugars Easy to Ignore?

Based on my experience and hundreds of conversations with Type 2 diabetics, I have learned the biggest reason diabetics often let blood glucose levels drift high—and remain high—is the lack of immediate negative feedback from their bodies.

High blood sugars are subtle and can be hard to identify until they reach a high and unhealthy point. With normal blood glucose levels in the 75-to-105 mg/dl range, what happens when your blood sugar gets up to 120? What do you feel? *Nothing.*

How about 140? Still nothing. What about 160? 180? You still feel normal. How can you be sick if you feel normal?

Maybe at 200 mg/dl or higher you might feel just a little off. You can't put your finger on it, but you just don't feel great. By the time your blood sugar gets to 300, you usually can feel it. It feels like you might be getting the flu. You're not sick but you feel just a little under the weather. Even then, you're in no *immediate short-term* danger so you'll tend to not treat it seriously.

But it is serious, and you need to know why so many diabetics regret their inattention or indifference to high blood sugars years later.

The Consequences of Long-Term High Blood Glucose

When I talk about the consequences of long-term high blood glucose, what do I mean? Long-term is totally dependent on the age and physical condition of a person when he or she is diagnosed with diabetes. For example, it stands to reason that a newly diagnosed young, Type 1 diabetic is starting his or her life as a diabetic with a healthier circulatory system, healthier kidneys, and a healthier heart than a newly diagnosed 60-year-old Type 2 diabetic.

What that means is that the young person has more time to learn about dealing with diabetes and to develop the habits he or she needs to live a long and healthy life. It's better for the young person to learn quickly but a slower adaptation is likely going to be less damaging to a younger diabetic than to an older diabetic.

Older Diabetics Must Act Quickly.

The older Type 2 diabetic does not have the luxury of taking a lot of time to change habits. A few years of high blood sugars for someone in their 40s, 50s, 60s, 70s, or 80s can have a very negative impact on health and survivability, whereas a few years of higher-than-ideal blood sugars for a younger person will not have as significant an impact.

This is a problem that must be taken seriously by people diagnosed with diabetes later in life. If you're diagnosed with Type 2 diabetes or as a borderline diabetic, you don't have the luxury of years before you need to start changing your habits. You need to begin acting now.

The Glucose Control Diet© is your answer to both losing weight and avoiding or reversing Type 2 diabetes. You will be amazed and pleased at both the immediate and lifelong impact of changing your food choices. When that change is combined with a slightly more active lifestyle, you're on your way to a healthier, diabetes-free life.

Although there is little *immediate* danger in periodic high blood glucose, there certainly are very severe long-term consequences with consistent high blood glucose over extended time. Consistent high blood sugars will contribute directly to circulatory problems—which in the long term will lead to heart problems, kidney problems, vision impairment, and even blindness, foot problems, and even amputations.

Consider these problems, not as *what will happen to you, but rather as what can be avoided or reversed by applying the Glucose Control Diet™*.

I would not be overstating if I were to say to all diabetics, pre-diabetics, or borderline diabetics that lowering your blood glucose levels and committing to keeping those levels normal is going to make the difference between living a long, healthy life or a short, unhealthy life.

We've talked about what we put in our mouths and how it all converts to glucose. Now let's talk about how we can use that glucose a little more effectively before it gets stored as fat.

Chapter 11

Modest Increases in Activity will Accelerate Your Weight Loss

Walking—A Great Lifelong Activity
The Trick with Life Is to Make It Look Easy.

—anon—

Two lifestyle changes are important for anyone who wants to lose weight and enjoy better health:

1. **Embrace Glucose Control Eating©.** This is by far the more important of the two lifestyle changes. You now have the information you need to start Glucose Control Eating©. Begin applying it now and you will be amazed at how much better you'll feel in short order.
2. **Embrace a slightly more active lifestyle.** Notice I said *"slightly."* Whatever additional activity you embrace, it must be within your capability to maintain. The key to maintaining your new activity level is not to start with much more than you're doing right now but gradually increase.

Daily Activity
Based on blood glucose testing and resulting insulin demand, if I do well in the first of the healthy lifestyles (eating) but am sedentary and don't walk the rest of the day, my blood glucose and therefore insulin demand is about 20% higher, which translates to a modest incremental weight gain. I use the word "modest" here because I'm referring to only one day.

You can lose weight without adding walking or other activity to your daily life, but if you add increased walking, you will lose weight faster, you will improve your mobility, your posture, and your appearance. You'll not only have a longer life, but you'll have a longer, healthy life.

This chapter is about stepping up the activity level in your daily life in ways you may never have thought of and making those new levels of activity your new active lifestyle. As you will see, increasing daily activity is an easy lifestyle change to make and easy to develop into a habit. I'll teach you how to start this new lifestyle while recognizing that many of you reading this book may have some significant limitations on what you can do now, so start slowly and build from there.

Why So Many European and Asian Nationalities Are Slimmer Than Americans

Over the past 40 years, I've visited urban and rural areas in about 60 countries on six of the world's seven continents—I haven't been to Antarctica—and have come to realize that most of the world's people walk a lot more than Americans do. Some may say that we Americans are lazy. I disagree totally with that premise. How much people of different countries walk is because of factors far out of the control of most of the world's citizens—primarily the historical development and design of cities and the economic imperatives of countries—that determine whether people walk a lot or don't walk much.

Most European and Asian cities were far along in their development hundreds of years before automobiles and trucks replaced carts drawn by horses, oxen, and humans as the primary vehicles for moving goods and promoting commerce. The widths of the streets in Europe and Asia were designed to accommodate the needs of the time. Buildings were built hard on both sides of narrow streets with little room for more than sidewalks and slow-moving carts.

Widening streets for automobiles in many big European and Asian cities is now prohibitively expensive and destructive of cities' infrastructure. As a result, the narrow streets remain unaccommodating to automobile driving and parking. The result: people walk or ride bikes.

On our first visit to China in 1980, our interpreters stated that Beijing had only 800 privately owned cars in the whole city of nine million people at that time. The rest of the motor vehicles were small trucks, taxis, and army vehicles. The result: millions of people walked or rode in a rolling sea of bicycles on every main street. Now Beijing has more than 20 million people with more than a million cars crawling in a perpetual traffic jam. But because of the economic imperative of general poverty, millions of people still walk and ride their bikes.

In Paris, London, Rome, Prague, Seoul, and many other large European and Asian cities the sidewalks are bustling and flowing with walkers. Walking is necessary, of course, but also enjoyable for native citizens and visitors alike. Only Manhattan, in American areas, comes close to matching the walking requirements and experiences of European cities.

A few years ago, we spent a month in the African country of Malawi volunteering at an orphanage started by two longtime friends, Tom and Ruth Nighswander.

This is an example of an economic imperative. Malawians have few cars and insufficient discretionary income to even dream of purchasing a car or fuel. Walking is the primary form of transportation and commerce. My mind's eye clearly recalls tall, slim, erect Malawian women walking in single lines with wooden branches, sacks of maize and jugs of water balanced firmly on top of their heads. This is the commerce of rural Malawi. This is their transportation system.

As you can guess, people in the areas I've just described are largely slim and healthy looking. Other factors may influence their slim appearance, but I believe walking is a significant contributor. The balance of this chapter will give you techniques to develop a pattern of walking more and making that pattern your lifelong habit.

Buy a Pedometer and Some Good "Around-Home" Walking Shoes

I recommend that you buy what I call "around-home walking shoes." Most of your walking is going to be around home, around the yard, around your neighborhood, visiting, shopping, and doing errands. Buy shoes that you're comfortable wearing for those purposes.

I also recommend buying a pedometer. Almost any sporting goods or outdoor store will have one and most are less than $15. You can also get more elaborate digital pedometers or fitness watches, but you don't need the more expensive one to get started.

The pedometer will measure with good accuracy how many steps you take in a day. For the most accurate results, you should attach it to a belt or the waist of your pants or skirt.

Once you get a pedometer it's important to keep a log of how many steps you're taking. Begin by establishing your baseline—how many steps you're taking now. It's best to do that for at least a week since some days, especially weekends, may vary from weekdays. Then use that baseline to compete with yourself. Each day try to beat the previous day's steps. After you've used it for a couple of weeks or so and have an idea of what you are doing and what you may be able to do in terms of steps per day, then you can start thinking about goals.

Here are some things to think about in your daily steps' goal setting. Dr. Catrine Tudor-Locke published a study in 2004 involving 200 men and women. The men in the survey took an average of 7,192 steps a day and the women in the survey took an average of 5,210 steps.

In 2001, the US Surgeon General, Dr. David Satcher issued "The Surgeon General's Call to Action to Prevent and Decrease Overweight and Obesity." The report recommended 30 minutes a day of moderate activity.

Most health experts seem to agree that 8,000 to 9,000 steps a day is an excellent healthy pattern to be in. That may sound daunting but I'm willing to bet that most of you will be surprised at how many steps you're already taking.

Whether your baseline is 1,000 steps a day, 3,000 steps, 5,000 steps or more, this suggestion is easy and very flexible. At the end of the first month, you'll not only feel healthier, but you'll also enjoy a feeling of physical pride that you may not have felt for a while.

Find a Friend to Walk with On a Regular Schedule

Finding a friend or friends to walk with is one of the best ways to build a regular walking habit. You'll have both company and commitment. You'll see things in your own neighborhood you never noticed from your car. You may end up stopping and talking to people who have lived near you for years but who you've never shared a story or even a greeting with. People who have enjoyed this habit for a long time talk about this time as a pleasant, satisfying part of their day.

Here are two stories of people in their upper 70s who have developed a habit of walking and maintained that habit for years—and all are healthy and trim.

My Sister, Rosanne, and Her Walking Friends

Eighteen years ago, my sister, Rosanne Bader, retired after 32 years as a teacher and principal in the Pomona Unified School District—now a board member of both Pomona Valley Hospital and Mount San Antonio Community College. She started walking with her friend and neighbor, Dona Avila, a retired art teacher in the same school district. Once they retired, the two ladies committed to starting a walking program together.

They live just two houses apart at the top of a hilly area covered with nicely spaced homes fronted with cedar and foothill pines surrounding the bigger oak, alder, and cottonwood trees. For nine months of the year flowering plants decorate their walks.

They made some early and lasting decisions about their walks that have served them well. They decided upon morning walks. "We start at 8 a.m." said Rosanne. "We agreed to a Monday-through-Friday schedule and we simply call each other the night before if a morning meeting or commitment requires a cancellation of the day's walk," she added.

Now 18 years later, Rosanne has new walking partners and talks warmly about her and Dona's lifestyle habit. "Since our homes are at the top of the hill, we always started out downhill. We liked to talk as we walked. At first, we could only talk on the downhill half. Coming home uphill we just walked without talking—not because we didn't want to talk, we just couldn't walk uphill and talk at the same time." "Within a short time," she says, "we could talk the whole way."

"It's just fun" she declared. "We greet our neighbors, wave to the cars and pick up trash along the way. The 2.2 mile up and downhill walk seems to go by so fast."

A two-mile downhill and uphill may very well be too difficult a starting point. Whatever you do, don't make your starting point too long or too hard. Make it easy enough that when you finish, you'll look forward to doing it the next day.

The Anchorage Trash Fairies

About nine years ago we moved to a new neighborhood, a few miles from where we had lived for more than 35 years. Early in the morning as I was leaving for work, I would often see a group of cheerful, physically fit neighbors walking, talking, laughing…and picking up litter. I knew some of them and asked how long they had been doing their early morning excursions. Judy Sedwick, apparently one of the leaders, said, "Well, I started when my daughter was in kindergarten and now my daughter's 43." Wow!

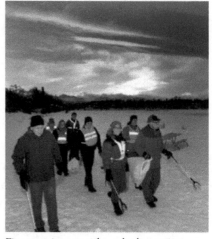

Five mornings a week—whether spring, summer, fall, or winter for about 40 years— this sociable and fit group of Anchorage citizens have been walking our neighborhood and picking up trash.

Not only have these folks stayed in good shape but they've had fun and made our little part of the world better.

The Importance of After-Dinner Walking or Similar Activities

At no other time in your day will activity have as much impact on your blood glucose and weight as the hours between dinner and bedtime. This is the time our promises die. This is the time our health gets superseded by sloth and TV…unless we actively choose health. This is not just other people's problems. It was mine too for a few years and it may be yours now.

In the early 1990s, I was approaching 50 and I noticed a more sedentary after-dinner pattern showing up in my life during the winter months. The summer months were not a problem because of the long daylight hours in Alaska. I would almost always be active and busy during those long, sunny summer evenings. More than once I recall my wife saying, "Rick, you'd better stop cutting the lawn. It's almost midnight and you'll disturb the neighbors."

For a couple of years, though, November through February was a different story. I found myself doing what I never thought I would do—surfing the television channels from about 9 p.m. to 11 p.m.

It didn't take me long to realize I was not only wasting two hours of my life each night, but I was also increasing my blood glucose by about 20%. Remember, increasing blood glucose means gaining weight. It didn't increase because I was eating more. It increased because I was burning less of the glucose I had put into in my bloodstream.

After gaining weight and getting a little softer around my stomach, I decided to make a simple lifestyle change. I decided I would try to get at least 15 to 30 minutes of some activity between dinner and bedtime.

After beginning that activity, my blood glucose not only went down during and slightly after the activity, but it also continued going down for a couple of hours even after I went to bed.

My Experiments with Blood Glucose and Weight Reduction from Modest After-Dinner Activity

After I first began to associate my after-dinner activity with a lowering of blood glucose even when I was sleeping, I decided to try an experiment to prove or disprove the premise that a relatively small amount of activity after dinner and before bedtime can have larger than usual impacts on blood glucose and weight reduction.

I decided the best way to establish the impact or lack of impact of activity after dinner was to eat the same or very similar dinners on consecutive nights and follow those dinners with either activity or inactivity before bedtime. I chose a dinner that I would eat often and made a special point of eating similar portion sizes.

It turned out my premise was valid.

When I followed my similar meals with 15 to 30 minutes of some activity after dinner as simple as walking around the block, walking to a neighbor's home, or riding my bike around the neighborhood, I found that about eight units of insulin was sufficient to balance that dinner. If I sat down in front of my computer or our TV set between dinner and bedtime and had virtually no activity, it would take about 10 units of insulin to balance the blood glucose my dinner had created. That's a moderate reduction in insulin demand and weight loss resulting from that modest activity between dinner and going to bed.

That reduced insulin demand meant less work for my pancreas and less weight gain—or weight loss—for the same meal.

That Small Amount of Activity Over a Year Translates into a Large Weight Loss

Let me explain the impact of that activity in another way. The roughly two units of additional insulin I needed to take when I had no activity after dinner is about the same amount of insulin I would take to balance a standard-size Hershey bar, which is a little more than 200 calories. Not having any activity after dinner was like adding the equivalent of a candy bar to my dinner.

Having no activity after dinner every day for a year is like adding 365 candy bars to your calorie intake. If you assume a candy bar is about 200 calories, that's roughly 75,000 calories' impact over a year. Every pound of fat is equivalent to about 3,500 calories which means those 75,000 additional calories —because of post dinner inactivity— would add over 20 pounds of fat per year.

The positive way to view that math is that those 15 to 30 minutes of moderate activity would mean a loss of about 20 pounds of body fat over a year.

Continuation of Fat Burning When You're Asleep

Now conventional wisdom would say that 30 minutes of light to moderate activity is insufficient to burn 200 calories, but conventional wisdom hasn't been tested like this. My observation is that a continuation result of calorie burning takes effect and a slight increase in metabolism continues prior to bedtime and for the first hours or more of your sleep.

My conclusion is based on the specific measurement of glucose reduction. That's why I've concluded that some activity between the time you eat and the time you go to bed is the *most important and effective activity you will have all day.*

It's a habit I've continued for years and you'll find it an easy action to start and an enjoyable habit to continue.

The first thing you need to do is to get into the mindset of moving after dinner. If you're one of those folks who gets up from the table, moves to the living room and positions yourself in front of a TV or a computer, changing that pattern and adding about a half hour of some physical movement after dinner will have a big impact on your weight and health.

So how do you get into the habit of doing this?

After-Dinner Activity Suggestions

1. Do some of your daily "out of home" chores after dinner instead of doing them before dinner. For example, do your food shopping and any other shopping or errands after dinner and when you do it, park farther away from the store than you normally would.

2. Instead of doing yard work on weekends, do a little bit each evening after dinner.

3. Get in a habit of taking an after-dinner walk with friends or your spouse or partner. It doesn't have to be long. It can be just around the block to start and let it build naturally to longer walks if you choose. This is different from a morning walk. It doesn't have to be as long to be effective in reducing the glucose created by your dinner.

4. If you go out to eat in a location that accommodates walking, get in the habit of parking three or four blocks away from the restaurant and walking to the restaurant. That action means you'll walk before you eat, and more importantly, after you eat.

5. If you have a shopping mall nearby, go there and walk around for a while.

6. When you do sit down in front of the TV, make it a point to get up and walk around your house or yard during commercials. This will also help you curtail snacking because a commercial break is one of the most common snacking cues.

Conclusion

You don't have to have to work hard after dinner, just move. You're going to move naturally after breakfast and lunch, but you don't necessarily move after dinner. You should begin this pattern and make it your habit. You will be astounded at the difference this will make in your weight and health over the years.

Lightning Source UK Ltd.
Milton Keynes UK
UKHW022022060622
404005UK00009B/2052